D1527945

# Guide to Program Evaluation for Physical Therapy and Occupational Therapy Services

**Evelyn Machan Andamo, MPA, OTR,**
is Chief of Rehabilitation Services
at the University of California
Irvine Medical Center
and Clinical Associate in their
Department of Physical Medicine
and Rehabilitation.

# Guide to Program Evaluation for Physical Therapy and Occupational Therapy Services

Evelyn Machan Andamo, MPA, OTR
EDITOR

The Haworth Press
New York • London

The Haworth Press, Inc.
28 East 22 Street
New York, New York
10010-6194

EUROSPAN/Haworth
3 Henrietta Street
London WC2E 8LU England

**Library of Congress Cataloging Publication Data**
Main entry under title:

Guide to program evaluation for physical therapy and occupational therapy services.

Includes bibliographical references.
1. Physical therapy—Evaluation. 2. Occupational therapy—Evaluation. I. Andamo, Evelyn Machan. [DNLM: 1. Hospital Departments—Organization & Administration. 2. Hospital Departments—standards. WX 223 G946]
RM701.G85      1984      362.1'78      84-8962
ISBN 0-86656-261-3

Printed in the United States of America

*To colleagues*
*and*
*future therapy administrators*

# Contents

# Contributors

**Catherine Erickson Barrett, MS, OTR,** is Director of Therapeutic Activities at Indianapolis Jewish Home, Inc. (Hooverwood), Indianapolis, Indiana. She is Adjunct Associate Professor of Occupational Therapy at Indiana University School of Medicine, Indianapolis, Indiana.

**Melva Diamante, MBA** in Labor-Management Relations, is Director of Employment at Memorial Sloan-Kettering Cancer Center, New York City, New York. She also teaches at Baruch College, City University of New York, and New York University. She is Vice President, Professional Development of Women in Human Resource Management.

**Harold J. Egli, MS, PT,** is manager of the Section of Rehabilitation Medicine at Geisinger Medical Center, Danville, Pennsylvania. He was former president of Medical Rehabilitation Directors and Coordinators, Inc.

**Jan Harrington, BS, RPT,** is Supervisor of Therapy at the Visiting Nurse Association, Colorado Springs, Colorado.

**Stephen Morgenstein, MS, RPT,** is in private practice with Midland Physical Therapy Group, Inc., Cranston, Rhode Island. He was formerly the Chief of Physical Therapy Department at Dr. Joseph H. Ladd Center, Exeter, Rhode Island.

**Diana L. Severs, BSHS, MBA,** is Management Engineer of Management Services at Geisinger Medical Center, Danville, Pennsylvania.

**Peter M. Synowiez, MHA** in Financial Management, is Administrative Director of Administration at Geisinger Medical Center, Danville, Pennsylvania.

**Michaele Tovar, MA, OTR,** is Supervisor of Occupational Therapy Department at University of California Irvine Medical Center, Irvine, California.

**Michael P. Weber, MBA, OTR,** is Senior Occupational Therapist at Ancorra Psychiatric Hospital, Hammonton, New Jersey. He is the founder of the Occupational Therapy Microcomputer Club.

**Zona Weeks, PhD, OTR, FAOTA,** is Associate Professor of Occupational Therapy at Indiana University, School of Medicine, Indianapolis.

# Foreword

Program evaluation has been around for some time; it has always been an important administrative tool. However, it has never been as *necessary* as it is today. We are not only in a dynamic, rapidly changing world, as the editor acknowledges, but in a world where major legislative changes are resulting in *legally fixed funding levels,* in the name of prospective, all-inclusive per diem rates.

We are entering an era in which a health care system will *truly* operate largely upon *fixed* resources. This is extraordinarily different from the fee-for-service reimbursement system of the past one and one-half decades, when the "more-you-do-the-more-you-get" (reimbursement) approach and philosophy prevailed.

Program evaluation is now necessary for survival, rather than academic fulfillment or "progressive administration," as was true during the 70s. Entire regions, states, counties, and, indeed, medical centers will be evaluating their programs in an effort to determine which program or its component contributes the most (in patient care outcome) in the most cost-effective manner; simply put, what activity generates most patient benefit for the least amount of resources.

Those clinical service administrators (diagnostic *or* therapeutic) who recognize the importance *and* the necessity for program evaluation will do their professions a service. That occupational and physical therapy administrators are recognizing the need to write about this absolutely essential activity will ultimately prove to be an inherent building block for the future of occupational and physical therapy professions. These professions seeing the reality of health and medical care, in terms of national (and tax-funded) priority in the 1980s and beyond, and recognizing the absolute requirement of effective programmatic evaluation, will combine to be the resultant team that is more of a health care *system*—for the future—than that we have known up until now.

William G. Gonzalez, MBA, MPA
Director, University of California
  Irvine Medical Center
Senior Lecturer, School of Management
University of California, Irvine

# Introduction

This book was conceived primarily for therapy service administrators, supervisors, and students in occupational/physical therapy administration—the administrators of the future. The selected readings compiled in this book offer insight and guidelines for one of the most important tasks in therapy services administration—program evaluation. While considering some of the most important issues, it does not claim to include all the necessary writings on therapy services program evaluation.

In this book, the therapy services program is a set of activities performed in a therapy department to attain its objectives utilizing managerial, technical, financial, and human resources. This set of activities may include staff continuing education, staff functions, treatment intervention, and/or equipment utilization. This concept illustrates the wide range of activities in therapy services program.

Evaluation, on the other hand, is the basic element for all the various functions of an administrator. It is a method by which judgments or conclusions are reached to pursue an action. Results of evaluations are the data base used by therapy administrators in order to plan, budget, organize, staff, direct, and coordinate their service. These evaluative results, therefore, are the catalysts for change and bases for action. Evaluation is an inherent element in the daily performance of therapy administrators. It provides them with information on the effectiveness (attainment of expected outcome) and efficiency (within the given resources) of the entire therapy services program or its various components.

Therapy services program evaluations may be classified into two categories, formal and informal. Formal therapy services program evaluation includes such activities as measurement of the impact of the department's therapeutic program, cost-benefit of staff continuing education, and effectiveness of a treatment approach. Supplies and equipment monitoring, comparisons of expenditure statements and past experiences, employee performance evaluations, and peer review are examples of informal evaluations. These evaluations are differentiated from the formal evaluations in that only the latter apply scientific methodology in reaching reliable and valid conclusions.

The various therapy services program evaluations presented in this book are either formal or informal, or a combination of both. Their commonality lies in the precipitants that demand program evaluations. Three of these are of utmost importance: (1) a super-industrialized environment; (2) finite resources; and (3) strong consumer advocacy groups.

Therapy services exist in a dynamic rapidly changing world—a super-industrialized environment! Without evaluations, the determination of critical activities which needs the administrator's attention becomes a difficult task. Time and effort will be diluted in various directions, and may be focused on less critical yet more time consuming activities. Crisis management occupies the administrators' time. They are busy struggling with bottle-necks leaving no time for program development. They are then unable to keep pace with the tempo of the environment in which the department has to survive. Program evaluation is the necessary catalyst which will assist therapy administrators in adapting to a rapidly changing world. They will be able to act rather than re-act.

Legislation is continuously being passed in Congress which points to the reality that the United States' resources are finite. Health care costs continue to outstrip inflation. Consequently, various health service providers are competing for federal, state, insurance company, and other private group dollars. The therapy administrators will have to evaluate the effectiveness of their services. These have to be maximized within the limited resources available. In light of scarcity, maintenance of cost curtailment efforts and heightened staff productivity need monitoring. Waste has to be minimized and energy efficient techniques adopted. These ecological approaches to health care management can be developed and maintained by therapy administrators with the aid of program evaluations.

In the surge of public interest advocacy groups in the United States, patients are no longer the passive health care consumers of the past. Therapy services have to be responsive to patient demand for accountability. This is enforced via governmental agencies such as the Joint Commission of Accreditation of Hospitals (JCAH) and other accrediting bodies. They provide administrative regulations and health consumer protection to ensure that the patients' therapy needs are adequately met in a cost efficient manner. Program evaluations will assist therapy administrators to identify areas of non-compliance with the regulatory requirements and barriers to high quality patient care so that corrective action may be undertaken.

Effort was made to incorporate articles that offer the most current and valuable approaches in response to the described precipitating forces. The purpose of providing the selected readings is to assist therapy administrators in implementing program evaluations.

In the first article, Weeks presents an overview of program evaluation in assessing therapeutic and support services. She also provides suggestions for design and implementation of specific program evaluations.

Morgenstein describes the development of a quality assurance program with a peer review-audit system as its primary component. The program incorporates the use of problem oriented record system (PORS). The potential for success of the program is measured by carrying out an external peer review audit.

Egli, Severs, and Synowiez's comprehensive departmental analysis utilizes a monthly productivity monitoring of patient charges as data base. This process links staffing allocation, equipment utilization, and revenue generation.

Diamante demonstrates a design for conducting management and staff performance assessment. The process is characterized as having four supportive and progressive steps. Each of the steps is discussed in detail and its crucial element is emphasized.

A method for assessing treatment philosophies is developed by Harrington. Two treatment philosophies, educational versus direct services, are compared using a retrospective chart audit-patient interview.

In the sixth article, Weber's use of microcomputers in therapy services program evaluations is explored within a traditional cyclic framework of planning—implementation—evaluation—correction. He compares various microcomputers with respect to their suitability for program evaluations. Finally, he offers salient points in the purchase of microcomputers and software for this purpose. A glossary of terms is provided at the end of this article to clarify the technical jargon.

Tovar depicts a multifaceted approach to equipment utilization analysis. The various data necessary in the analysis are provided at length. Corrective actions resulting from the analysis are discussed to reiterate the value of the analytical process.

The eighth article by Barrett is a presentation of the clinical education program directors' responsibility in ensuring competency levels of occupational and physical therapy clinical students. The article portrays a methodology in evaluating clinical education programming to meet this responsibility. Furthermore, it indicates that this evaluation will enhance the body of knowledge and quality of service in the disciplines of both the academicians and clinicians.

The articles may be read in any preferred sequence or one may select to review any single topic of interest since each is self-contained and provides sufficient information for implementation.

At this point, I would like to acknowledge and express my gratitude to the many people without whom this venture could never have metamorphosized into a book. I cannot say enough to thank Sara Bernstein, whose valuable comments and suggestions enhanced this book. I would also like to express my sincere appreciation to the University of California Irvine Medical Center for its continued encouragement and support. I am also grateful to Penny L. Temple and Joanne McClancy, who expertly typed and proofread the final manuscript, and to Ethel Ross, my Administrative Assistant, who provided me with secretarial assistance. I also would like to give thanks to my husband, Manny, who was most supportive of women's emancipation. Finally, I give thanks to Evaleen, Emmalyn, and Emmanuel III, my children, who weathered through my stormy moods during this venture.

*Zona R. Weeks,* PhD, OTR, FAOTA

# 1   Program Evaluation: The Process for Accountability

## INTRODUCTION

Occupational and physical therapists are familiar with the process of patient/client evaluation, which helps provide appropriate treatment and post-discharge planning. Fewer therapists are accustomed to thinking in terms of program evaluation. Many have made no provisions for the periodic review of their own administrative and treatment procedures to assure efficient and effective use of personnel, facilities, and material.

There has been much discussion in recent years about "accountability," the concept of therapists being accountable for their actions. The term has been used in reference to the treatment process, but seldom in reference to the support systems that are essential for effective treatment programs. Administrative procedures, in-service learning experiences, staff qualifications and morale and other factors all affect the end goal of patient/client improvement. Therefore, if one can understand the functioning of the entire operation, its strengths and weaknesses, one can determine the needs of that operation in some areas while demonstrating cause for confidence in other areas.

Since the first concern of therapy programs is quality of patient/client care, the results of an evaluation should provide useful information to judge the present value of services to clients and to aid in decision-making for changes in the program. Thus, whether the clients see the evaluation results or not, they are as much a part of the "audience" served by a program evaluation as are the therapists providing the services, the administrators, and insurance companies benefiting from more cost-effective service for their clients. The occupational and physical therapy professions at large also benefit from program evaluations, since evaluations provide assessments of the value of professional services and a basis for comparison with other programs. If administrative procedures are streamlined and treatment becomes more effective, funds expended for an evaluation might soon be recovered. More efficient operation and improved self-image could in themselves make the expenditure worthwhile.

This paper attempts to direct the thinking of occupational and physical therapists toward consideration of program evaluation. It does not provide a final complete design for evaluation of a specific program; rather, it makes suggestions and provides ideas from which specific program evaluations may be designed.

## PROGRAM AND PERSONNEL STANDARDS

Standards must be used to decide whether a program and its personnel are functioning at satisfactory quality levels. Certain standards, criteria, and guidelines are available in the occupational and physical therapy professions against which programs and personnel can be compared. Standards of practice for occupational therapy services have been approved by the American Occupational Therapy Association.[1,2] Guidelines describing responsibilities of "entry level assistant" and "entry level therapist" have also been adopted by the American Occupational Therapy Association.[3] The American Physical Therapy Association has adopted and published standards of practice for physical therapy services and physical therapy practitioners.[4,5] By these means, the profession delineates conditions and standards of performance that are believed to be necessary for quality service and patient care. Comparisons can also be made with facilities offering similar services, if they are willing to share evaluative and other records. It is not enough that administrators or staff therapists think their treatment program is valid; standards guide and provide a means to systematically judge efficiency and quality of service.

## PROGRAM EVALUATION PURPOSE AND SCOPE

Administrators and the evaluator should jointly establish the purpose, or purposes, of a program evaluation. Examples of purposes for an evaluation may include: to make informed decisions regarding existing or proposed programming, to determine direction for change, to compare current status with national standards and professional and community developments. Is there something specific about the departmental functioning that needs to be studied, or is there a vague feeling of disquiet about the total program, with unidentified problems? The purposes or reasons for doing a program evaluation relate to the scope of the evaluation. Some aspects of a program that could be evaluated include treatment delivery procedures, scheduling methods, student programs, budget in relationship to cost effective services, written reporting methods and forms in use. The scope or range of the evaluation will depend, then, upon the identified purposes, the priorities of the questions or problems needing analysis, budgetary constraints, and staff availability, among other factors. The administrator and staff, working together, may be able to define and limit the evaluation to conform to unavoidable restrictions.

A number of factors must be considered when thinking of developing an occupational or physical therapy program evaluation. First, one must consider what would be entailed in the design of the evaluation. Let us say that an evaluation is being considered for a multi-faceted occupational or physical therapy service in a general hospital serving adults and children with physical dysfunction, both in- and outpatients. Staff levels include registered therapists, certified assistants, and aides. The evaluation model for such a department could be modified for other departments serving patients/clients with any type of physical or psychosocial dysfunction.

Evaluation in this effort might be defined as the process of systematically determining one or all of the following: 1) the value of services provided to patients/clients, 2) the efficiency and effectiveness of administrative procedures, 3) the competency of personnel, and 4) the value of the student program. Such a definition of what this evaluation is expected to determine appears simple until the realization occurs that decisions of quality and value must be based on measurable objective standards and valid judgments acceptable to the profession. The general purpose for this type of program evaluation might be stated in the following manner: to assess quality of direct services and support functions.

## HOW TO SELECT AND PREPARE FOR A PROGRAM EVALUATOR

Care must be taken in selecting an evaluator, since as mentioned earlier objectivity is of utmost importance. If the sponsor of the evaluation (person or agency requesting the evaluation or funding it) chooses an evaluator with a conflict of interest interfering with his judgments, results of the evaluation are unlikely to be accepted by knowledgeable persons. An experienced evaluator should know how to maintain objectivity and fairness by ethical standards evident to those being evaluated. He should also be aware of possible sources of error in an evaluation, such as "halo effect," initial impression, stereotyping, rating tendencies or errors, and his own biases.

There are many occupational and physical therapy programs

which, though needing evaluation, will not be able to provide funds for an outside trained evaluator to come in and study the program. Before deciding that money cannot be budgeted, however, consideration should be given to the benefits that might result from an evaluation.

Experienced program evaluators can be found in schools of education of many large universities, as they have taken on the task of educating people for this responsibility. Lack of familiarity with treatment facilities, however, might necessitate pairing this type of external evaluator with an experienced occupational or physical therapist, who may not be an expert on program evaluation, but who certainly can answer the evaluator's questions on clinical aspects of the program. The national occupational and physical therapy associations have for many years provided a type of program evaluation for professional education programs in their accreditation procedures. Teams visit educational programs for purposes of evaluating them through prepared self-study documents, interviews, and so forth. The writer believes that a need exists for similar teams to be available to clinical facilities. It is not expected that the national associations could fund these teams, or even necessarily provide them. Rather, private teams of experienced therapist-evaluators could be formed and utilized on a consultancy basis.

If an external evaluation consultant is not practical, a person from the facility (an "internal evaluator") may be utilized. A person from the facility knows the program and would not need to take time to study certain features already familiar to him, but he must attempt to control subjectivity and biases. Emotional involvement with the program might prevent valid assessment. An internal person may coordinate collection of much of the relevant data and organize the data into a form which could be shared with knowledgeable outside consultants before final judgments and decisions are made by those within the facility. An internal evaluator can be a therapist or administrator from within the department, or a capable person from another department or level of the facility who can be allowed time for the responsibilities.

The evaluator may wish to know the program objectives before beginning the study. At times, the evaluator may decide to do a "goal free" evaluation. He measures whatever outcomes are present, regardless of what is stated in the goals and objectives. The need of an external evaluator should be determined before he arrives so that all is in readiness to begin. An evaluator must be given office space in which to work, and the equipment, material, and personnel support needed to do the job. Both secretarial help and the assistance of some professional persons to collect data may be needed.

Consideration must be given to the projected use of the data results, and the relevance of the planned study to current functioning. Will the evaluation be wide-ranging enough to provide important information, yet concise enough to be manageable? If values are used in judging the evaluation results, will those values be acceptable to the persons being evaluated so that the judgments are credible? If the values are fair interpretations of the values of the profession, there should be little question of acceptability. Will the person making the judgments (evaluator, administrative decision-makers, and/or other selected persons) be considered impartial and capable of reaching objective conclusions?

What questions will the evaluator be expected to answer, and how valuable will that information be? Such questions might include the following:

1. Are goals and objectives and their priorities reasonable?
2. Are administrative procedures adequate? Are forms appropriate and useful?
3. Are the therapists and other personnel satisfactorily prepared to treat the types of conditions referred?
4. Do patients/clients benefit from the treatment used?
5. Are appropriate treatments administered by qualified staff?
6. Is there an adequate in-service program?
7. Is the student program satisfactory?
8. What are the attitudes of significant persons to the treatment and functioning of this department?
9. Is morale good?

To make the response to these questions objective and measurable, two types of response sheets can be designed: 1) criteria sheets for those doing the evaluation to mark when matching program standards to standards defined by national occupational or physical therapy associations, and 2) scale-type response sheets requiring ratings of various factors by staff, students, patients/clients, physicians, and others. A numerical rating scale from excellent to poor could be used, or an agree-disagree form could be used in response to statements regarding quality of aspects of the program. In addition, space for comments should be provided.

## DISSEMINATION OF RESULTS

Prior to beginning an evaluation, decisions must be made regarding the publicity to be given to this evaluation. Will a newspaper announcement be made to inform the public of funds to be spent? Who is to be informed of the purpose and results of the evaluation, and how are they to be informed? Is the public entitled to know the results of the evaluation, as consumers of the service or as taxpayers supporting public institutions?

An outside evaluator and the sponsor may wish to have a contract delineating the evaluator's role and the persons or groups to whom the results are to be disseminated. Such a contract should prevent later disagreements about who has a right to the results. It should be understood who has the right to make the report public, or if it is to be made public. The contract should also specify the persons with authority to edit the evaluation report, with safeguards for the evaluator against gross report changes with which he disagrees, but with provisions for the sponsor to indicate any major disagreements with the results. Plans for future program re-evaluation to assess changes instituted and progress made since the original evaluation results may be incorporated in the report.

## DEVELOPMENT OF COOPERATIVE EFFORT

Either the facility administrator or the occupational or physical therapy department director may seek the program evaluation. In any event, responsible persons must agree that an evaluation would be helpful; their mutual support plus cooperation from various participants to be questioned and studied is necessary for a successful evaluation effort. To gain cooperation, participants must first be informed of the intent of program evaluation, that of determining where and why there are strengths and weaknesses in program components, without blaming individuals for any deficiencies. The assumption should be that all persons are performing in the manner they believe is best, and that if the evaluation demonstrates that certain procedures are ineffective, they will be open-minded enough to consider alternatives. Anxiety and "cover-ups" can be avoided if everyone involved attempts to be open and supportive. Trust must be established among the personnel, administrative decision makers, and the evaluator.

An initial meeting should be held to inform personnel of the nature of the evaluation. This initial meeting is meant to explain and to provide an opportunity for those most directly involved to ask questions and voice concerns. Involved personnel have a right to know in what ways evaluation results might influence administrative decisions and policies.

A tentative schedule for the evaluation sequences should be developed jointly by the evaluator and the sponsors. Together they can determine how long it will take to obtain and analyze data, and prepare a final report. For example, they may decide that one week is necessary for initial interviews, evaluation of physical plant, and other preliminary examinations, another week for examining all reports and records, another week for in-depth interviews and observations, and a final week for any additional data collection and preparation of a report.

If this is a first-time evaluation, there are probably no procedures or policies to guide the evaluation. Prior to his arrival, an experienced evaluator may be able to suggest some guidelines, to which a committee of facility personnel may wish to add policies. Succeeding evaluations should become smoother in operation as pitfalls are discovered and documented. Once the various evaluation procedures are learned, a department's personnel should be more aware of what to look for in effective functioning, thus improving their ability to engage in self-evaluation.

During the evaluation, lines of communication must be established between the evaluator, the administrative decision-makers, and the personnel. The evaluator needs to know what is expected in terms of protocol in such things as obtaining records, calling personnel from their duties for interviews, and informing administrators of plans to visit other departments, etc. Persons who wish to contact the evaluator at times other than those scheduled should know the procedure for contacting the evaluator for an appointment or where to send written communications. Those providing data need to be assured of anonymity, if necessary. Security of personnel information must be maintained, and all data should be kept confidential by the evaluator until the final report is submitted.

Department personnel assisting the evaluator in obtaining data or in other processes, should be appointed and allowed time away from job duties so that they can perform the tasks required. Such assistants might need special training to learn methods of helping the evaluator collect data. If so, someone should be designated to teach collection and recording techniques.

## EVALUATING THE EVALUATORS

The people involved in an evaluation want the assurance that the results will be fair to them and free of bias. Perhaps the personnel would like to select an impartial panel of knowledgeable persons from the profession to review the evaluation methodology, data, and findings. These persons would, in effect, be evaluating the evaluator. If the panel agrees with the evaluator's findings, the personnel should have greater confidence in the results, since more extensive judgment has focused upon the data.

If certain departmental personnel feel that some of the results are not valid, they should have an opportunity to state reasons why they question the results. For example, they may believe that the evaluator observed a component of the program only during an unusual day. Although the staff might be expected to challenge criticism more than praise, the staff might welcome critical evaluator statements. For example, critical comments may help the staff obtain budgetary support for a program component that is ineffective because of insufficient funds, or they may indicate a need for another staff person.

## METHOD OF EVALUATION

A number of evaluation experts have developed frames of reference for evaluating programs. Most do not lend themselves in unmodified form to evaluation of occupational or physical therapy programs. For illustration, ideas have been borrowed from the Provus Discrepancy Evaluation Model,[6] the Stufflebeam CIPP Model,[7] and Stufflebeam's Administrative Checklist for Reviewing Evaluative Plans.[8]

### Program Components for Evaluation

Figure 1.1 shows a suggested sequential method for carrying out an evaluation. First, the components of the program to be evaluated must be determined. These can be global components such as administrative and treatment processes, or more specific ones, such as certain administrative sub-functions (for example, inventory procedures) or certain treatment sub-sections (as a stroke rehabilitation group, or a self-care program).

### Necessary Information for Judging Components

Once the components to be evaluated are determined, thinking focuses on what information is needed to judge each component. The evaluator's presence at the facility being evaluated is imperative to gather information for most evaluations, unless the evaluation is an incomplete study of forms or some particular data not requiring on-site visitation. Evaluation of administrative components would require studying such factors as 1) reports, records, and the forms on which they are filed, 2) available space, equipment, and supplies, 3) amount and administration of budget, 4) diagnoses of patients being treated, 5) various administrative procedures (as inventory, staff meetings, and supervision methods), 6) organizational structure, 7) communication procedures within and outside the department, 8) personnel information (such as professional-non-professional staff ratio, patient-staff ratio, staff turn-

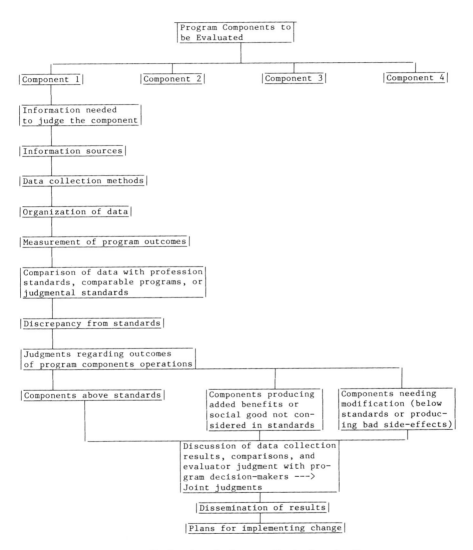

**Figure 1:** Evaluation design: method of evaluation.

over rates, and peer supervisory review procedures), and 9) student programs.

Evaluation of treatment components would include some of the above administrative information relative to staff functioning, budget, and factors pertinent to patient/client treatment.

## Information Sources

In addition to interviews of various individuals, personnel records and job descriptions need to be examined to analyze personnel competency in relation to services provided (staff members' educational background, post-graduate training, work record, etc.). Monthly reports and annual reports can be used for information on diagnoses and case load. Progress reports are useful in studying methods of reporting patient treatment and thoroughness of care. All forms can be studied for effectiveness of written communication within and outside of the department.

## Data Collection Methods and Organization

The evaluator might use checklists, rating scales, or observation methods to gather some data important to patient/client treatment. He might formally or informally observe the treatment procedures, morale, attitudes, and rapport of staff and patients/clients. He might wish to inspect patient/client screening, measurement, and reporting forms. Philosophy, rationale, and objectives for the treatment program may be studied. Review of charts and progress reports is important. Interviews of appropriate administrators, directors, staff, and other facility personnel, and clients might be required.

Collection of these data requires a plan of action to make collection, storage, and retrieval of information efficient. Consolidated forms for recording and summarizing data may need to be designed for the initial and subsequent evaluations.

Some systematic method of collecting and organizing the data needs to be devised. Sampling procedures can be used to scale down the collection of certain types of data to manageable size. For example, not all records need to be examined and not all patients/clients need to be interviewed. Organization of the data may be by means of special forms or by summary paragraphs. The desired form for the final evaluation report and its uses should also be considered.

## Program Outcome Measurement

Measurement of program outcomes should be possible through use of the data results. It should be possible to compare the results to standards of practice defined by the national occupational and physical therapy associations. Comparison with other similar programs might be desirable, and the evaluation results should make this practical. At times, only judgmental standards of authorities in the profession or in administration can be applied for comparison. This involves expertise and common sense. Some parts of the program may be obviously ineffective in terms of cost benefit ratio, or better methods in use may become clear when examined on paper.

## Discrepancy Delineation and Judgment

Discrepancies from standards should be thoughtfully delineated and recorded. When results are examined in full, judgments regarding operations of various program components can tentatively be made. Certain components will be above standards, while others will be shown to produce side effects not easily compared with standards. Other components will be seen as needing modification if results do not show compliance with minimum standards or if undesired side effects nullify any possible benefits. An evaluator may prefer to avoid making judgments from the obtained data on outcomes, leaving that to the facility, or he may prefer to work with facility decision-makers to jointly check the accuracy of the data and develop judgments.

## Implementation of Dissemination Plan

Decisions regarding dissemination of results should have been made before the evaluation began. Personnel from the department being evaluated and any affected administrators should be informed as soon as possible of the results. Outsiders and news media should be notified in the manner and in a time sequence deemed best. The evaluator may request adherence to contractual agreements requiring designated distribution, or if an evaluation was done solely for the self-improvement of a department, there may be no requests for dissemination of results. Only portions of the final report may need to be shared with interested persons or agencies (such as information regarding the benefits of part of a program for certain diagnostic conditions). The form of the final report may be at the discretion of the evaluator, or sponsors of the evaluation may request that it be made in a specific form.

## CONCLUSION

Although it is pleasant to hear good things about one's program in evaluation results, the purpose of the effort is not for self-satisfaction, but rather to allow for examination of the program to see objectively where it is effective and where it is not in terms of operation and service. The information gained is intended to be useful in planning for change. Clear visualization of where the program needs modification should motivate action.

## SUMMARY

Demonstration of accountability for administrative and treatment aspects of a therapy services program is expected of occupational and physical therapists. This paper represented an attempt to encourage occupational and physical therapists to engage in program evaluations to provide evidence of accountability. Program evaluations provided mechanisms for determining program strengths and weaknesses and bases for sound planning. Use of professional standards and comparison with other programs were offered as guidelines to consider in judging the value of a program. An overview of the process of program evaluation to assess quality of therapeutic and support services was provided, along with suggestions for designing and implementing specific program evaluations.

## NOTES

1. American Occupational Therapy Association, "Standards for Occupational Therapy Service Program," *American Journal of Occupational Therapy*, 1969, 23:81–82.

2. American Occupational Therapy Association, "Standards for Occupational Therapists Providing Direct Service," *American Journal of Occupational Therapy*, 1973, 28:237.

3. American Occupational Therapy Association, *Entry Level Role Delineation for OTRS and COTAS*. (Rockville, Md.: American Occupational Therapy Association, 1980).

4. American Physical Therapy Association, *Standards for Physical Therapy Services and Physical Therapy Practitioners*. (Washington, DC.: American Physical Therapy Association, 1980).

5. American Physical Therapy Association, *Competencies in Physical Therapy: An Analysis of Practice*. (San Diego, Calif.: Courseware Inc., 1977).

6. M. M. Provus, *Discrepancy Evaluation*. (Berkeley, Calif.: McCutchan Publishing Corp., 1971).

7. D. L. Stufflebeam, W. J. Foley, W. J. Gephart, E. Guba, R. L. Hammond,

H. O. Merriman, and M. M. Provus, *Educational Evaluation and Decision-Making.* (Itasca, Ill.: Peacock Publishers, Inc., 1971).

8. D. L. Stufflebeam, "Meta Evaluation," *Occasional Paper Series Number 8.* (Kalamazoo, Mich.: Western Michigan University Evaluation Center, 1975).

# BIBLIOGRAPHY

Ellingham, C. T., and Fleischaker, K. "Competencies in Physical Therapy. A Resource for Written Self-Assessment and Clinical Performance Evaluation and a Component of a Department's Quality Assurance Program." *Physical Therapy*, 1982, Vol. 62, No. 6, 845–849.

Morgenstein, S., Simpkins, S., and Maring, J. "Development of a Quality Assurance Program as an Integral Part of the Physical Therapy System." *Physical Therapy*, 1982, Vol. 62, No. 4, 464–469.

Worthen, B. R., and Sanders, J. R. *Educational Evaluation: Theory and Practice.* Worthington, Ohio: Charles A. Jones Publishing Co., 1973.

*Stephen S. Morgenstein,* MS

# 2 Quality Assurance Program and Peer Review as Its Primary Component

## INTRODUCTION

Providing high quality care to all persons receiving services has long been the goal of the physical therapy profession.[1] Defining what is meant by "high quality care" and how best to monitor its implementation and outcome has been an ongoing process.[2,3,4,5] Over the past 10 to 15 years this process has received further impetus from government agencies and consumer groups. By 1977, standards for developing a quality assurance program had been delineated by the American Physical Therapy Association.[6]

The development of standards for evaluating the quality of health care should take into account three frames of reference described by Nicholls:[7]

- the focus of the standards
- determination of national data to be collected, and
- direction of action to be taken to assure high quality.

Structure is the framework that provides for the actual provision of care and includes laws and regulations; processes are the actual behaviors involved in providing care and can be expressed in the form of protocols or regimens; and outcomes are the results of these behaviors.

For a quality assurance program (QAP) to be successful, a therapy service has to be amenable to the evaluation of its structure, processes, and outcomes. The mere presence of regulations and protocols does not, as Reibel[8] pointed out, automatically ensure quality care. The effects of this care (outcomes) must be evaluated. The peer review audit system is an effective way to evaluate outcomes.

The author wishes to gratefully acknowledge Ms. Joyce Maring, PT and Ms. Joan Flynn, PT for their assistance in editing this paper and Ms. Lisa Marrapese for her assistance in the preparation of this manuscript.

The purpose of this paper is to describe the development of a QAP based upon the problem oriented record system (PORS) and having a peer review record and treatment audit system as its primary component. The program described in this article was developed at a state-run residential facility (Facility X) for approximately 800 people with developmental disabilities. At the time that this program was developed, there were eight registered physical therapists (one being the chief of the department and two others, supervisors) and 10 physical therapy assistants employed by Facility X.

## DEVELOPING THE QUALITY ASSURANCE PROGRAM

The philosophy upon which the QAP was based was that high quality care is what each person receiving services deserves and expects to receive. Staff members believed this and wanted to work towards realization of the goal of providing high quality care.

Administrative support for this philosophy and the QAP was sought and obtained. This was imperative since several components of the QAP (most prominently, the audit system) removed staff from their

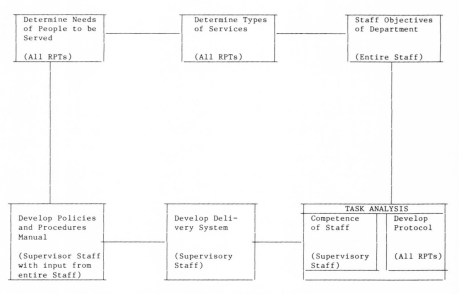

**Figure 2.1:** Quality assurance program development process. Reprinted from *Physical Therapy* (62:464–469, 1982) with the permission of the American Physical Therapy Association.

revenue generating tasks (i.e., evaluation and treatment). In Facility X, the therapy administrators were always trying to fill vacant staff positions. The recruitment and retention of staff were difficult tasks because salaries were less than those offered in the private sector, few opportunities existed for professional advancement, the disabilities of the people receiving services were severe, and there were few opportunities for continuing education. It was emphasized that the development of a QAP with the staff interaction and educational component inherent in peer review would, to some extent, help make the staff retention and recruitment tasks easier to accomplish.

Knowledge of quality assurance theories and programs was gained by the supervisory staff since they were to be primarily responsible for the development and implementation of the QAP. Review of the literature, observation of QAP's already in place in other facilities, and attendance at continuing education programs were ways in which this knowledge was obtained. Encouraging members of the staff who had knowledge in QAP's to share that knowledge with their peers was helpful in promoting staff acceptance of the program.

Once the above steps were undertaken, the development of the specific (QAP) began (Figure 2.1).[9] The process of development was cyclical in nature. The QAP was based upon the needs of the people to be served. A data base with guidelines and significant negatives as described by Feitelberg[10] was developed to serve as the basis of the needs assessment (Figure 2.2). An analysis of the significant negatives appearing most frequently on the data bases helped us to determine the specific needs of the people to be served. After developing the needs, we identified the types of services necessary to meet these needs. These services included:

- sensorimotor integration and gross motor development programs
- training in the activities of daily living (such as eating)
- chest physical therapy
- provision of corrective shoes and adaptive equipment, and
- continual evaluations to monitor changes in function.

A task analysis[11] was then carried out to determine the classification of staff needed to provide these services and to begin the development of protocols and treatment regimens. The most effective systems for delivering these services (i.e., direct provision by a staff member or indirect provision by a parent, caretaker, etc.) were developed next. Finally, the departmental policies and procedures manual was developed. This manual described which services were to be provided, how and by whom. Using this manual to document the standards made

| WNL | ABN | N/E | | |
|-----|-----|-----|---|---|
| | | | 1:00 | Profile and history |
| | | | 2:00 | Observation of general condition and level of responsiveness |
| | | | 2:10 | Communication |
| | | | 2:20 | Behavior |
| | | | 2:30 | Medications |
| | | | 2:40 | Bowel and Bladder |
| | | | 3:00 | Specific evaluations of anatomical and physiological systems |
| | | | 3:10 | Skin and soft tissue |
| | | | 3:20 | Cardiovascular |
| | | | 3:30 | Pulmonary |
| | | | 3:40 | Skeletal and articular. There are no skeletal abnormalities. Note skeletal implants. Significant Negatives: decrease of joint motion caused by structural limitations, absence of parts. |
| | | | 3:50 | Muscular. Voluntary muscle control is within normal limits. Significant Negatives: deficits in strength, length, bulk; abnormal tone. |
| | | | 4:00 | Neurological examination |
| | | | 4:10 | Visual function |
| | | | 4:20 | Gross sensorium. Neuromuscular and sensorimotor systems are intact. Significant Negatives: deficits in cranial/peripheral nerve function, incoordination; dyskinesias; decreased proprioception and kinesthesia; deficits in the sensations of touch, pressure, stereognosis, two-point discrimination, and temperature. |

**Figure 2.2:** Data base and examples of the data-base guidelines. WNL = Within normal limits; ABN = Abnormal; N/E = Not evaluated. Reprinted from *Physical Therapy* (62:464–469, 1982) with the permission of the American Physical Therapy Association.

these standards an integral part of the department and easily accessible to the staff required to implement them.

To help ensure that each staff member had a vested interest in the QAP, its development was participative in nature. This approach to program development and supervision, outlined by Hickok[12] and implicit in the work of Payton and associates[13] necessitated that supervisory personnel be mature enough to allow for such an educational experience to take place.[14] A system of meetings was used to promote this approach (Figure 2.3). This system allowed for an exchange of ideas, comments and suggestions, and provided a mechanism for the continued review of each step in the development of the QAP. In addition, the system allowed for the involvement of the entire staff in the development of the audit system.

# DEVELOPING THE PEER REVIEW AUDIT SYSTEM

If the goal of high quality care is to be achieved, the results of the services being provided must be assessed. This can only be done effectively if there is a system in place which has a defined set of guidelines. The PORS is such a system:

Step I:   The Problem-Oriented Record

    A.  Data Base and Data Base Guidelines
    B.  Initial Evaluation in the SOAP format
    C.  Flow Sheets
    D.  Progress Reports in the SOAP format
    E.  Discontinuation Reports in the SOAP format

Step II:   The Audit Process

    A.  Record Audit
    B.  Treatment Audit
    C.  High Frequency Record Audit

Step III:   The Educational Programs

    A.  Discussion between auditor(s) and clinician(s) being audited after the audit has been completed.
    B.  Re-Audit process and correction of discrepancies
    C.  Physical therapist group discussion of audit results held at least four times a year.

For an audit system to be effective, two conditions must be met. First, the system's objectives must be to aid in the development of a

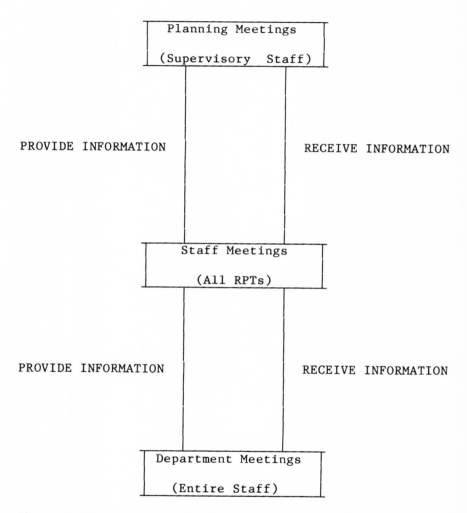

**Figure 2.3:** Mechanism for facilitating participative supervision and program management.

more competent clinical staff. The audit system must not be used as a mechanism for administering discipline. Second, the audit system must be developed with the involvement of the entire staff (i.e., all personnel who are to be audited). As mentioned before, the system of meetings was helpful to this end.

The reader is referred to Feitelberg's work[15] for a definitive explanation of the steps outlined. The patient's treatment chart, developed in the fashion of a problem oriented record, was audited for completeness, analytical sense, reliability, and efficiency (C-A-R-E) on the part of the clinician treating the patient. Egan[16] believes that this record audit is an "explicit audit based on a comparison of the components of a completed record with a set of predetermined standards." The standards developed will be different for each facility. Facility X emphasized written documentation. This resulted in the need for the staff to document in more than one section of the patient's medical chart. This propensity for documentation was illustrated in the audit form (Appendix A).

In addition to the traditional record audit, a treatment audit (Appendix B), and a high frequency record audit (Appendix C) were also developed. The purpose of the treatment audit was to observe whether or not a clinician's hands-on skills was on par with his or her knowledge as demonstrated by the record audit and vice versa. A treatment audit is an "implicit audit because, in the absence of a simple correct approach to treatment, auditors must give opinions concerning the appropriateness of care based not on predetermined criteria, but on consensus of peers having similar knowledge and experience."[17] As a result, an additional benefit of the treatment audit was to provide an opportunity for the exchange of ideas about treatment approaches.

Before the audit system was initiated, a workshop on peer review and the audit process was presented by a quality assurance consultant recommended by the American Physical Therapy Association. All therapists attended this workshop. Record and treatment audits were then conducted by two member peer review teams. Peer review team audits were done of records and treatments of all staff including the supervisory staff. Staff served on the peer review teams on a rotating basis. This allowed for therapists with different educational, experiential, and clinical backgrounds to work together and therefore resulted in greater potential for professional growth. The work of each therapist was audited by his or her peer at least once every two months. A record audit took approximately one hour, and a treatment audit took approximately 45 minutes. An additional 30 to 45 minutes were needed for the discussion between auditors and the clinician who had been audited. A peer review audit committee, comprised of two members of the supervisory staff, developed the rotation and audit schedules.

The determination of which patients were to be audited could have been made by random selection; by request of the therapist (due, for example, to a particularly difficult case); by diagnosis or by disability. At Facility X, the first two methods were used.

The audit team completed the record audit prior to observing the treatment. This gave the members of the team insight into the need of the person being treated and an idea of the techniques and approaches to be used by the clinician during the treatment audits.

The high-frequency record audit (HFRA) was a shortened form of the record audit used by the peer review teams. The items selected for the HFRA were those thought by the supervisory staff to be most ethically, legally, and professionally significant. The HFRA allowed several records to be audited in less time than it would take to audit one record using the long form; it provided supervisory personnel with a survey tool. The HFRA was used to get an overview of how well the needs of the people receiving services were being met and how well staff members were complying with the PORS.

## THE EDUCATIONAL PROCESS

The educational process flowed directly from the audit system. Figure 2.4 outlines this process which was based upon the auditor's analysis of the information gathered during the audits and their ensuing discussion with the clinician who had been audited.

The record and treatment audit forms were designed to encourage this analysis and discussion. The auditors were required to write a narrative summary of the audits and to make recommendations including whether or not a re-audit was indicated. This analysis and discussion would have the potential to improve the record keeping and/or treatment abilities of the clinician who has been audited. This clinician was required to comment on the findings of the auditors.

The analysis and discussion portions of the audit were carried out in a private setting with the forms being kept in record files of the clinician who had been audited. The clinician was responsible for recording in a peer review audit book the name of the patient who was audited, the date of the audits, and whether or not a re-audit was recommended. The peer review committee used this information to monitor how well the staff was keeping to the audit schedule.

As the experience with the peer review audit system grew, it was evident that criteria needed to be developed to determine when a re-audit was indicated. Using the system of meetings as the forum for discussion, a set of guidelines was developed identifying "major" versus "minor" deficiencies. A "major" deficiency indicated that a re-audit was necessary. Examples of "major" deficiencies included "No" checks for:

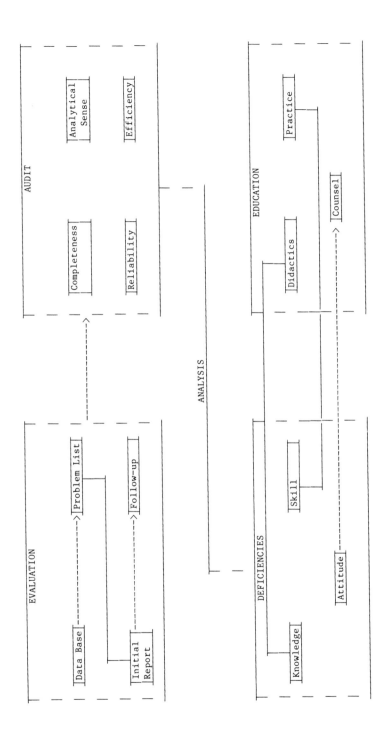

**Figure 2.4:** Educational process.

- any section or subsection of the treatment audit, and
- section II, subsection A, letters "d" or "e" of the record audit.

The other letters in the subsection of the audit with a "No" checked were considered to be "minor" deficiencies.

The use of these guidelines was tempered with the exercise of professional prerogative and common sense by the auditors. This was especially important since staff shortages necessitated that caseloads be exceedingly high. The use of professional prerogative was reflected in the fact that deficiencies in the areas of "secretarial" tasks (e.g., filing details) and adherence to time frames were not looked upon as critically as they would have been had the staffing shortages not been present. Deficiencies in the areas of knowledge, skill, and/or attitude were, however, looked upon as being quite critical and educational programs were set up to correct these deficiencies.

When deficiencies in knowledge were uncovered, the clinician was given a number of ways to correct them. Included in the resources available were: (1) articles from journals which had been collected and indexed over the years; (2) a medical library; (3) a departmental library; (4) the libraries of several universities (one of which had a medical school library); (5) departmental and interdepartmental inservice training programs; and (6) continuing education programs.

Deficiencies in skill necessitated practice in the area of weakness. This practice took place under supervision of staff members proficient in those areas. Those staff members were not necessarily supervisory personnel.

If problems such as deficiencies in record keeping and/or patient care went uncorrected even after participation in educational programs, counseling was done by the clinician's immediate supervisor. The purpose of the counseling was to promote open communication between the clinician and his or her immediate supervisor so that the underlying causes of the problem(s) could be identified and eliminated. If necessary, supervisory personnel could become involved but only after staff at the preceding administrative and professional levels had failed to correct the problem(s).

Once deficiencies had been identified and the potential sources for correction made available, the re-audit was done to determine if they had been corrected, or if further remedial action was indicated.

Therapist staff meetings were held quarterly to examine and discuss the common deficiencies, needs and problems which were identified during the previous period's audits. The discussions were kept general in nature and ways were sought in which to meet these needs and solve these problems. When appropriate, the results of these meetings were shared with other staff members. One example of a need which was identified related to the writing of the Subjective-Objective-Assessment-Plan (SOAP) reports. Both therapists and assistants were having difficulty determining what information should be included in the "objective" section. In addition, therapists were repeating objective findings when all that was needed was reference to a flow sheet which already included these data. The solution to this problem was to review the procedures for writing SOAP reports at a staff inservice. Re-audits after the inservice revealed that, for the most part, these reports were now being written properly.

## ASSESSING THE QAP

Once the QAP was in place and the peer review system was functioning, the staff needed to step back and see if the QAP was serving the purpose for which it was designed. To this end, the structure, process, and outcome standards which were developed for evaluating the quality of care at Facility X were examined.

An external peer review audit of the structure standards was done by an expert in quality control. This person was selected from a list of resource people developed by the American Physical Therapy Association and had no affiliation with Facility X or any member of its staff. It was this person's judgment that the structure of the QAP had the potential for promoting high quality care.

The results of the record and treatment audits showed that people receiving services were demonstrating improvement in those functional tasks which had been identified on evaluation as being their areas of weakness (i.e., mobility, eating, and/or social interaction). These positive outcomes, while by no means the result of a controlled scientific study, were taken from flow sheets which contained objective data and pointed to the possibility that the process standards (protocols and regimens) were appropriate.

The QAP pointed to several potential areas for research: (1) the comparison of the success of various treatment techniques; (2) the comparison of the quality of the clinician's written documentation with the results of his or her treatment programs; (3) the development of criteria for determining prognosis based on functional diagnosis; and (4) the development of time frames for achieving short and long term goals in the areas of functional activities such as mobility.

The major objective of the physical therapy department was to provide high quality patient care (e.g., to improve the functional abilities of the people being treated). To the extent that there were indications that this objective was being met, the QAP had been successful.

## SUMMARY

The development of a QAP must be founded on the philosophy that each person being treated expects and is entitled to receive high quality care. Administrative support for this philosophy and knowledge of the theories of quality assurance are necessary if a QAP is to be successful. A participative approach to program development is essential for promoting acceptance of the program.

A system of meetings served as a mechanism for fostering this approach and as a forum for continued review of the QAP. This allowed the QAP to remain dynamic in nature.

The QAP must be based on the needs of the people to be served and take into account the three frames of reference for setting standards to evaluate the quality of health care. These standards must themselves be amenable to assessment. Therefore, a system such as PORS must be utilized.

A component of the PORS was a peer review audit system which was effective in monitoring the outcomes resulting from process and structural standards. Both record and treatment audits were designed. A potential for research can be found in correlating the results of record versus treatment audits (e.g., is a therapist who keeps good records necessarily a good clinician?). The audit system served as the basis for the educational component of the QAP and was not used for purposes of administering discipline.

To determine if the QAP was functioning as designed, an external peer review audit was done. The questions to be answered by this type of audit include:

- do the protocols reflect state-of-the-art knowledge and practice?
- are the people being treated getting better?, and
- is the structure of the QAP such that it allows for alteration of the QAP as indicated by the clinical experiences of the staff and the needs of people being served?

The process for developing the QAP and the peer review audit system described herein is applicable to other agencies wishing to formulate such programs.

## NOTES

1. *Standards for Physical Therapy Services and Physical Therapy Practitioners* (Washington, DC: American Physical Therapy Association, 1978).

2. A. M. Egan, "Peer Review: One Department's Experiences," *Physical Therapy*, 1979, 59:877–880.

3. A. B. Hightower, and J. W. Griffin, "Peer Review: An Adventure in Real Life," *Physical Therapy*, 1974, 54:943–948.

4. O. D. Payton, S. Seubott, G. DeFlora et al., "Quality of Patient Care and Peer Review System: A Model," *Physical Therapy*, 1970, 51:296–300.

5. R. P. Noland, "Components of Quality Health Care," *Physical Therapy*, 1970, 50:34–39.

6. *Competencies in Physical Therapy: Analysis of Practice* (San Diego, Calif.: Courseware, Inc., 1977).

7. M. E. Nicholls, "Terminology in Quality Assurance," in *Nursing Standards and Nursing Process*, ed. M. E. Nicholls and G. Wessels (Wakefield, Mass.: Contemporary Publishing, Inc., 1977) 31–38.

8. J. S. Reibel, "Quality Health Care and the Federal Government," *Physical Therapy*, 1969, 49:366–372.

9. S. Morgenstein, S. Simpkins, J. Maring, "Development of a Quality Assurance Program as an Integral Part of Physical Therapy System," *Physical Therapy*, 1982, 62:464–469.

10. S. B. Feitelberg, *The Problem Oriented Record System in Physical Therapy* (Burlington, Vt.: Samuel B. Feitelberg, 1975) 21–28.

11. N. T. Watts, "Task Analysis and Division Responsibility in Physical Therapy," *Physical Therapy*, 1971, 51:23–25.

12. R. J. Hickok, "Participative Supervision in Physical Therapy," *Physical Therapy*, 1969, 49:731–734.

13. Payton, "Quality of Patient Care."

14. P. Hersey, K. Blanchard, *Management of Organizational Behavior: Utilizing Human Resources* (Englewood Cliffs, N.J.: Prentice-Hall Inc., 1977), 126–130.

15. Feitelberg, *The Problem Oriented Record System.*

16. Egan, "Peer Review."

17. Ibid.

Appendix A

PHYSICAL THERAPY
Record Audit

Client's Name _____    Living Area: _____    Social Security No: _____

|  | YES | NO | N/A |  |
|---|---|---|---|---|
|  |  |  |  | I. HEALTH SERVICES SECTION |
| a. (c) | ___ | ___ | ___ | A. Is there a prescription for therapy? |
| b. (c) | ___ | ___ | ___ | B. Has the prescription been renewed quarterly? |
| c. (c) | ___ | ___ | ___ | C. Is the prescription signed by the doctor? |
|  |  |  |  | ADDITIONAL COMMENTS: |
|  |  |  |  | II. PHYSICAL THERAPY SECTION |
|  |  |  |  | A. Data Base |
| a. (c) | ___ | ___ | ___ | a. Does the name of the person being evaluated appear on all pages of the Data Base? |
| b. (c) | ___ | ___ | ___ | b. Is the Data Base complete as indicated by responding to WNL, ABN, or N/E? |
| c. (c) | ___ | ___ | ___ | c. Is the Data Base dated and signed? |
| d. (c) | ___ | ___ | ___ | d. Is the collected data reliable? |
| e. (c) | ___ | ___ | ___ | e. Is good judgement shown in selecting which items to evaluate? |
|  |  |  |  | ADDITIONAL COMMENTS: |
|  |  |  |  | B. Problem List |
| a. (c) | ___ | ___ | ___ | a. Does every significant physical therapy problem defined from the Data Base appear on the Problem List? |
| b. (a) | ___ | ___ | ___ | b. Are new problems added to the Problem List when defined in the clinical record? |
| c. (e) | ___ | ___ | ___ | c. Are problem statements formulated clearly as the person's functional problems? |
| d. (e) | ___ | ___ | ___ | d. Is the problem solved in a reasonable amount of time. |
|  |  |  |  | ADDITIONAL COMMENTS: |

Form RA-2 (11/80)

Key: (c) completeness; (a) analytical; (r) reliability; (e) efficiency

Client's Name: _____

|  | YES | NO | N/A |
|---|---|---|---|

C.  Initial Report
    a.  Is the report titled, "Initial Report"?
    b.  Is the report SOAPed appropriately?
    c.  Is Objective information referred to the Data Base to avoid redundancy?
    d.  If the Data Base is incomplete, is there:
        1.  an explanation for why it had not been completed?
        2.  a plan for completion?
    e.  Does the initial Assessment take into account the total Problem list and the Subjective and Objective data?
    f.  Are there short term goals (STG) and long term goals (LTG) for each problem relating to physical therapy?
    g.  The goals:
        1.  are they logical in light of current data?
        2.  is the STG defined in terms of date of completion?
        3.  does the LTG follow from the STG?
    h.  Can the LTG be reached within one (1) year?
    i.  Is there a plan for each active problem relating to physical therapy?
    j.  Are plans structured in the following categories:
        1.  additional data?
        2.  specific management: frequency/type? by whom?
        3.  client/"family" education?
    k.  Is the Plan appropriate?
    l.  Is the referral to the Data Base for objective data done appropriately?
ADDITIONAL COMMENTS:

D.  Progress Reports
    a.  Are they written at least quarterly for direct programs and at least semi-annually for indirect programs?
    b.  Is each SOAPed appropriately?
    c.  Is each dated and signed?

a.  (c)
b.  (c)
c.  (e)
d.
    1.  (r)
    2.  (r)
e.  (a)

f.  (a,r,c)

g.
    1.  (a)
    2.  (a)
    3.  (a)
h.  (a)
i.  (a)
j.
    1.  (a)
    2.  (a)
    3.  (a)
k.  (r,a)
l.  (e)

a.  (e)

b.  (c)
c.  (c)

Form RA-2 (11/80)

33

Client's Name _____

| | YES | NO | N/A |
|---|---|---|---|

e. (e)   e. Do progress reports speak to all of the active problems that the treatment are trying to resolve?

f. (e)   f. Are deferred areas from the Data Base followed up?

g. (a)   g. Does the Assessment consider the total Problem List and the Subjective and Objective data in demonstrating good analytic sense of the problem?

h. (a)   h. Are differences in perception between the therapist and person being treated made explicit in the Assessment section?

i. (a)   i. Do the goals and plans get altered when appropriate?

j. (a)   j. Are the goals and plans clear?

k. (e)   k. Is there evidence of communication with other team members?

l. (a)   l. Is there evidence of discharge planning when appropriate?

m.   m. The goals:

1. (a)   1. are they logical in light of current data?

2. (a)   2. is the STG defined in terms of date of completion?

3. (a)   3. does the LTG follow from the STG?

n. (a)   n. Are the STG's being met?

1. (a)   1. If not, are possible reasons presented in Assessment?

2. (a)   2. Are actions to correct problems presented in Plan?

o. (a)   o. Can the LTG be reached within one (1) year?

p. (c,e)   p. Are appropriate incidental progress reports (shoe transactions, visits to orthopedic clinic, adaptive equipment transactions, impromptu consultations, etc.) in place?

q. (e)   q. Is the referral to flow sheets for objective data done appropriately?

ADDITIONAL COMMENTS:

E. Flow Sheets

a. (c)   a. Do flow sheets contain necessary administrative information, i.e. person's name, living area, and Social Security number?

b. (e)   b. Are the entries at least monthly?

c. (a)   c. Are appropriate parameters identified for a given problem either by selection of a pre-defined flow sheet or by entries onto a blank flow sheet?

Form RA-2 (11/80)

34

Client's Name _____

| | YES | NO | N/A |
|---|---|---|---|
| d. (r) | | | |
| e. (e) | | | |
| f. (e) | | | |
| g. (c) | | | |

d.  Are identified parameters followed through?
e.  Are flow sheets used where appropriate?
f.  Are flow sheets utilized to promote efficiency?
g.  Is each entry initialed and dated (including year)?
ADDITIONAL COMMENTS:

| | YES | NO | N/A |
|---|---|---|---|
| a. (c) | | | |
| b. (c) | | | |
| c. (c) | | | |
| d. (c) | | | |
| e. (c) | | | |
| f. (c) | | | |
| g. (c) | | | |
| h. (c) | | | |
| i. (c) | | | |
| j. (c) | | | |

F.  Discharge or Discontinuation Report
a.  Is there a Discharge or Discontinuation report if appropriate?
b.  Is the report titled appropriately?
c.  Is the report SOAPed?
d.  Is the Objective data written out?
e.  Is the report dated and signed?
f.  Does it include a statement of the current status of each active problem relating to physical therapy?
g.  Is there a statement of the level of goal attainment?
h.  Does it include clear plans for follow-up by a provider or "family"?
i.  Does it include a statement of client/"family" education?
j.  Is there evidence of transfer of records or verbal communication with a provider or "family"?
ADDITIONAL COMMENTS:

| | YES | NO | N/A |
|---|---|---|---|
| a. (c) | | | |

G.  General
A.  Has material been filed in the proper order?

Form RA-2 (11/80)

35

Appendix A (Cont.)

Client's Name _____

|  | YES | NO | N/A |
|---|---|---|---|

III. ACTIVE TREATMENT SECTION

A. Plan of Care

a. (e)    a. Is it part of an interdisciplinary plan? If it is not and it stands alone:

1. (e)    1. Is it up to date?

2. (a)    2. Is it problem oriented?

3. (a)    3. Do the STG and LTG reflect Assessment found in the Initial or Progress Reports?

4. (a)    4. Is the LTG one which can reasonably be reached within one (1) year?

5. (r)    5. Are the Procedures/How Recorded data accurate?

ADDITIONAL COMMENTS:

B. Monthly Providers Comments

a. (c)    a. Are they written when appropriate?

b. (e)    b. Are they in the record by the appropriate day?

c. (c)    c. If written by the therapist as the pivotal person on the interdisciplinary plan, do they describe consultation with other team members?

d. (r)    d. Do they speak to the program?

e. (a)    e. Do they assess the Subjective and Objective data to determine whether or not the Plan is successful?

ADDITIONAL COMMENTS:

Form RA-2 (11/80)

Appendix A (Cont.)

Client's Name _____

SUMMARY OF AUDIT:

RECOMMENDATIONS:

Auditor(s) Signature(s) _____

Date _____

COMMENTS FROM AUDITEE:

Auditee(s) Signature(s) _____

Date _____

RECOMMENDATIONS:

Form RA-1 (11/80)
Adapted from Medical Center Hospital of Vermont
Department of Physical Therapy – Patient Record Audit (Revised 5/78)

DR. JOSEPH H. LADD CENTER
PHYSICAL THERAPY
TREATMENT AUDIT

Client's Name: _____    Living Area: _____    Social Security No.: _____

| | YES | NO | N/A | |
|---|---|---|---|---|
| a. | | | | I. DISCUSSION PRIOR TO OBSERVATION OF TREATMENT |
| | | | | a. Does the therapist* know the following about the person being treated? |
| 1. | ___ | ___ | ___ | 1. approximate age |
| 2. | ___ | ___ | ___ | 2. precautions |
| 3. | ___ | ___ | ___ | 3. contraindications to treatment |
| 4. | ___ | ___ | ___ | 4. special problems |
| | | | | ADDITIONAL COMMENTS: |
| | | | | |
| | | | | II. OBSERVATION OF TREATMENT – SOCIAL |
| a. | | | | a. Is the therapist humanistic in approach? |
| 1. | ___ | ___ | ___ | 1. Is the person appropriately dressed or draped? |
| 2. | ___ | ___ | ___ | 2. Is there social interaction taking place? |
| 3. | ___ | ___ | ___ | 3. If there is, does it blend with the treatment? |
| 4. | ___ | ___ | ___ | 4. Does the therapist tell the person what is being done? |
| 5. | ___ | ___ | ___ | 5. Does the therapist explain to the person the "why" of what is being done? |
| 6. | ___ | ___ | ___ | 6. Does the therapist respect the wishes of the person regarding the treatment program? |
| | | | | ADDITIONAL COMMENTS: |
| | | | | |
| | | | | III. OBSERVATION OF TREATMENT – TECHNIQUE |
| a. | | | | a. Are transfers done safely? |
| 1. | ___ | ___ | ___ | 1. Is the person allowed to assist in transfers to the best of his/her ability? |
| b. | ___ | ___ | ___ | b. Does the therapist provide the appropriate amount of safety guarding? |
| c. | ___ | ___ | ___ | c. Do the techniques used seem appropriate in light of the goals set for the client? |

ADDITIONAL COMMENTS above

*"Therapist" may be RPT, PTA, PTPA, or any person carrying out indirect therapy program which is being monitored by an
RPT or PTA (e.g., teacher, IAMR, workshop staff member, etc.). Definition of "therapist" for each audit must be
indicated under I. ADDITIONAL COMMENTS above

Form TA-1 White (3/80)

Appendix B (Cont.)

Client's Name _____

|  | YES | NO | N/A |
|---|---|---|---|
| d. | ___ | ___ | ___ |

d. Does the therapist attempt to motivate the person to actively participate in the program:

ADDITIONAL COMMENTS

IV. DISCUSSION AFTER OBSERVATION OF TREATMENT

|  | | | |
|---|---|---|---|
| a. | ___ | ___ | ___ |
| b. | ___ | ___ | ___ |

a. Is the therapist able to give the rational for the treatment technique used in light of the goals set for the client?

b. Did the therapist and the person being treated accomplish what they wanted to during this treatment session?

ADDITIONAL COMMENTS:

Form TA-1 White (3/80)

39

Appendix B (Cont.)

Client's Name: _____

SUMMARY OF AUDIT:

RECOMMENDATIONS:

Auditor(s) Signature(s) _____
                        _____
                        Date

COMMENTS FROM AUDITEE:

RECOMMENDATIONS:

Auditee(s) Signature(s) _____
                        _____
                        Date

RE-AUDIT DATE:

Form TA-1 White (3/80)

40

Appendix C

DR. JOSEPH H. LADD CENTER
Physical Therapy
High Frequency Record Audit

Auditee: _____ Client: _____

| | YES | NO | N/A | YES | NO | N/A |
|---|---|---|---|---|---|---|
| **Prescription** | | | | | | |
| 1. (c) present | ___ | ___ | ___ | ___ | ___ | ___ |
| | | | | | | |
| **Data Base** | | | | | | |
| 1. (c) present and complete | ___ | ___ | ___ | ___ | ___ | ___ |
| 2. (r) correlates with Problem List | ___ | ___ | ___ | ___ | ___ | ___ |
| 3. (r) gives reason area is a problem | ___ | ___ | ___ | ___ | ___ | ___ |
| 4. (r) pick item and check it | ___ | ___ | ___ | ___ | ___ | ___ |
| 5. (a) All necessary areas screened | ___ | ___ | ___ | ___ | ___ | ___ |
| | | | | | | |
| **Problem List** | | | | | | |
| 1. (c) in front of Physical Therapy Section | ___ | ___ | ___ | ___ | ___ | ___ |
| 2. (r) problems relevant to physical therapy supported by information in Data Base Initial Report | ___ | ___ | ___ | ___ | ___ | ___ |
| 3. (a) sound judgement is used in defining problems | ___ | ___ | ___ | ___ | ___ | ___ |
| 4. (e) new problems are added to Problem List as appropriate | ___ | ___ | ___ | ___ | ___ | ___ |
| | | | | | | |
| **Initial Report** | | | | | | |
| 1. (c) present and S-O-A-P according to policies and procedures | ___ | ___ | ___ | ___ | ___ | ___ |
| 2. (r) problems demonstrate management by goals and plans | ___ | ___ | ___ | ___ | ___ | ___ |
| 3. (r) areas deferred from Data Base followed-up | ___ | ___ | ___ | ___ | ___ | ___ |
| 4. (a) Assessment, Goals, and Plans are appropriate and realistic | ___ | ___ | ___ | ___ | ___ | ___ |
| 5. (e) referral to Data Base for Objective data is done appropriately | ___ | ___ | ___ | ___ | ___ | ___ |
| | | | | | | |
| **Progress Report** | | | | | | |
| 1. (c) addresses all problems | ___ | ___ | ___ | ___ | ___ | ___ |
| 2. (r) Goals and Plans demonstrate follow-through by documentation | ___ | ___ | ___ | ___ | ___ | ___ |
| 3. (a) Assessment, Goals, and Plans are appropriate and realistic | ___ | ___ | ___ | ___ | ___ | ___ |
| 4. (e) problems solved in a reasonable amount of time | ___ | ___ | ___ | ___ | ___ | ___ |
| 5. (e) referral to flow sheet for Objective data is done appropriately | ___ | ___ | ___ | ___ | ___ | ___ |
| 6. (e) written quarterly (direct): semi-annually (indirect) | ___ | ___ | ___ | ___ | ___ | ___ |
| | | | | | | |
| **Flow Sheets** | | | | | | |
| 1. (c) entries at least monthly | ___ | ___ | ___ | ___ | ___ | ___ |
| 2. (r) identified parameters are followed through | ___ | ___ | ___ | ___ | ___ | ___ |
| 3. (a) parameters included are appropriate for problems being monitored | ___ | ___ | ___ | ___ | ___ | ___ |

Form HFRA-1 (11/80)

Key: (c) completeness; (a) analytical sense; (r) reliability: (e) efficiency

Appendix C (Cont.)

|  | YES | NO | N/A | YES | NO | N/A |
|---|---|---|---|---|---|---|
| **Discharge or Discontinuation Report** | | | | | | |
| 1. (c) present if appropriate | ___ | ___ | ___ | ___ | ___ | ___ |
| 2. (c) all Objective data is written out | ___ | ___ | ___ | ___ | ___ | ___ |
| 3. (r) demonstrates follow-through on all defined problems | ___ | ___ | ___ | ___ | ___ | ___ |
| 4. (a) management and status at discharge are logical in view of Assessment, Goals, and Plans | ___ | ___ | ___ | ___ | ___ | ___ |
| 5. (a) Plans for follow-up are appropriate | ___ | ___ | ___ | ___ | ___ | ___ |
| **Plan of Care** | | | | | | |
| 1. (c) present and up-to-date | ___ | ___ | ___ | ___ | ___ | ___ |
| 2 (a) LTG can be achieved in one (1) year | ___ | ___ | ___ | ___ | ___ | ___ |
| **Monthly Providers Comments** | | | | | | |
| 1. (c) present and written on time | ___ | ___ | ___ | ___ | ___ | ___ |
| 2. (r) speak to all programs | ___ | ___ | ___ | ___ | ___ | ___ |

SUMMARY OF AUDIT:

RECOMMENDATIONS:

Auditor Signature _____
Date _____

COMMENTS OF AUDITEE:

Auditee Signature _____
Date _____

Form HFRA-1 (11/80)

*Harold J. Egli, MS, PT*
*Diana L. Severs, BSHS, MBA*
*Peter M. Synowiez, MHA*

# 3 Developing a Productivity Monitoring System

## INTRODUCTION

Hospital costs continue to grow and health dollars continue to consume an even greater proportion of the Gross National Product. With this trend, the burden also grows to assure health care managers that they are getting the most out of the resources entrusted to them.

The Rehabilitation Medicine Department at Geisinger Medical Center, Danville, Pennsylvania, instituted a Productivity Monitoring (PM) system in an effort to deal with resource concerns. The department wanted assurances that the charges for their services were equitable in terms of costs to deliver them, and management wanted a method of evaluating the work load and staffing levels for the department. The PM system has been successful in meeting both of these needs.

The Geisinger Rehabilitation Medicine Department consists of Physical and Occupational Therapy Services under its direct aegis. A functional relationship exists with other member departments of the multidisciplinary team.

## BACKGROUND

A routine operational audit of the Rehabilitation Medicine Department by the Internal Audit Department in February 1981 raised questions about the relative value charging system then in use. (A system had been developed six years before, using best estimates of the staff.) The audit raised doubts about the validity of the relative values assigned to the various treatments. The audit also suggested that an ongoing productivity monitoring system could be useful in the management of the department and could be developed as a natural consequence of a new relative value system. In mid-1981 a request was made to the Management Engineering Department for assistance and direction in developing the system. The project was implemented upon approval of the request. The purpose of this paper is to describe the evolution of a productivity monitoring system for a rehabilitation medicine service including physical therapy and occupational therapy departments.

## OVERVIEW OF THE SERVICES

The Geisinger Medical Center consists of a 566-bed hospital with seventy-some specialty and subspecialty services offering tertiary care to the population of Pennsylvania and surrounding states.

The Physical Therapy Department consists of three treatment areas: hydrotherapy, therapeutic modalities, and the gym. The staff includes six full-time registered physical therapists and five full-time physical therapy aides. Student affiliates receive clinical training in the department for ten months of the year. Physical Therapy provides services for both inpatients and outpatients during the hours of 8 a.m. and 5 p.m. Monday through Friday, and 8 a.m. to 12 noon on Saturday. Care is provided for patients on inpatient units and in several outpatient clinics as well as in the treatment area. In fiscal year 1980–81 the service had 28,245 patient visits and provided 41,839 treatments.

The Occupational Therapy Service had 6,466 patient visits and provided 7,893 treatments. It consists of five professional personnel working five days per week, 8 a.m. to 5 p.m. Monday through Friday. The department's treatment areas contain an Activities of Daily Living evaluation and therapy room as well as two general treatment rooms.

## SYSTEM DEVELOPMENT

The process used by the management engineer in developing the PM system included the following steps:

- Preliminary staff meetings
- Data collection
- Data analysis
- System implementation and follow up

## Preliminary Meetings

Initial meetings were held by the manager of Rehabilitation Medicine and the management engineer with the responsible administrative officers and the chiefs of the Physical Therapy and Occupational Therapy Services to review the reasons for developing the PM system, the process to be used, the timetable for completion, and the results to be expected. After general agreement was reached on these points, the manager and the management engineer met with the staff of each service to review the plan and to provide more in-depth information as to the work required of the staff in the data collection phases.

## Data Collection

The following information was required to develop the new charging and PM systems:

1. Hands-on time, total time, and skill level* required to perform individual procedures.
2. Average workload volume for each department.
3. Work load distributions by time of day, day of week, and month of year.
4. Equipment usage, cost and depreciation rates.
5. Time required for non-patient care duties including team meetings, staff meetings, etc.

Procedure time and skill level information was obtained from several sources:

1. Flow process charts with time estimates by qualified staff members.
2. Observation by Management Engineering personnel.
3. Comparison with previous studies in other institutions.
4. Direct work load recording by staff members.

Work load volume and distribution data were obtained by the therapy staff's direct work and load records (see Figure 3.1), patients' service sheets, and the department's monthly accounting reports. An attempt to gain such information from the patient scheduling system failed due to inherent problems in this system. The department manager, service chiefs, and staff provided the necessary information regarding non-patient care duties.

An equipment list provided by the Accounting Department served as the source for equipment costs and depreciation rate data.

The direct work load recording was reported by staff over ten working days.

## Data Analysis for New Relative Value System

The previous relative value units used to assign patient charges were allocated according to *total* procedure time. This was not entirely appro-

*Skill level connotes educational background required of the employee performing the procedure.

Date _____

Treatment Area _____

| Patient Name | Patient Arrival Time | Patient Departure Time | Procedures Done | Therapist's Initials | Comments |
|---|---|---|---|---|---|
| | | | | | |
| | | | | | |
| | | | | | |
| | | | | | |
| | | | | | |
| | | | | | |
| | | | | | |
| | | | | | |
| | | | | | |
| | | | | | |
| | | | | | |
| | | | | | |
| | | | | | |
| | | | | | |

**Figure 3.1:** Rehabilitation Medicine work load data.

priate because of the differences in the intensity of individual procedures. For example, one 30-minute procedure (assisted exercise) may
require a full thirty minutes of staff time while another (hot packs) may
require only five minutes of staff time. To charge more equitably for
procedures, the proposed relative value system was developed using
total average direct procedure costs. There are two components for each
established cost, personnel and equipment. A sample calculation is
shown in Figure 3.2.

Personnel cost is the product of the average hands-on time (in
minutes) per procedure and the average personnel cost per minute.
Differences in personnel costs for different skill levels performing the
same procedure are taken into account.

Equipment cost per procedure is the depreciation cost per month,
divided by the average number of procedures performed per month
using the piece of equipment. When more than one piece of equipment
may be used for a given procedure, equipment costs are allocated
according to *total procedure time*. The total equipment cost is the sum of
all equipment.

The total average direct procedure cost is, then, the sum of the
personnel and equipment costs. The number of relative value units
assigned is the total cost divided by the cost of the procedure with the
lowest total cost in the service. Physical Therapy and Occupational
Therapy relative value units were calculated separately. Figures 3.3 and
3.4 demonstrate the direct procedure costing and recommended relative
value units (RVUs).

## Data Analysis for Productivity Monitoring System

Productivity is defined as the ratio of man-hours required to perform the
work at hand to actual man-hours worked. Calculation of required
man-hours should include the direct patient care hours required, a
coverage allowance for peak work load periods, and a constant time
allowance for indirect work load. The actual hours worked are obtained
from staff schedules; exclude all sick, vacation, holiday and educational
time; and include an allowance for breaks and personal time. To further
calculate required staffing levels, education, vacation, holiday and sick
time must be included. Productivity should be monitored on a monthly
basis and staffing requirements recalculated based on six-month aver-
ages. The forms used in the process are illustrated in Appendices A to F.

Direct work load is defined as time required to perform procedures
for which patients are charged. The relative value units used to calculate
this time are based on hands-on time and a coverage allowance of 25
percent of remaining total procedure time where applicable. The number of relative value units assigned to a procedure is the average time

1.  Direct Personnel Cost:

    a.  Minimum Assistance:        PT:   ( 4.0 min) x ($ .16/min) = $ .64
        (Requires Supervision     Aide: ( 1.0 min) x ($ .09/min) = $ .09
        to Minimal Assistance)

    b.  With Assistance:          PT:   ( 8.0 min) x ($ .16/min) = $1.28
        (Requires Assistance      Aide: ( 8.0 min) x ($ .09/min) = $ .72
        of two FTEs)

    c.  Prosthetic Training:      PT:   (31.0 min) x ($ .16/min) = $4.96
                                  Aide: ( 0.0 min)

    d.  Floor Patient:            PT:   (13.5 min) x ($ .16/min) = $2.16
                                  Aide: ( 0.0 min)

2.  Equipment Cost:

    a.  For equipment numbers 002, 003, 041, 314, 317, 318, 319 and 325, the
        depreciation cost (replacement cost ÷ depreciation rate) is $60.88.  The
        average number of procedures per month is 992, allocated as follows:

|                          | Number    | Minutes       | Avg. Minutes |
| Procedure                | Per Month | Per Procedure | Per Month    |
|--------------------------|-----------|---------------|--------------|
| (1) Minimum assistance   | 99        | 25.0          | 2475.0       |
| (2) With assistance      | 714       | 21.0          | 14994.0      |
| (3) Prosthetic training  | 30        | 51.0          | 1530.0       |
| (4) Floor patient        | 149       | 13.5          | 2011.5       |
| TOTAL                    | 992       |               | 21010.5      |

   $60.88 ÷ 21010.5 = $ .003/minute

   Average Equipment Cost Per Procedure (D x F)

   (1) Minimum assistance       .08        D = minutes per procedure
   (2) With assistance          .06        F = $ .003/minute
   (3) Prosthetic training      .15
   (4) Floor patient            .04

3. Total Cost ( = Sum of Personnel and Equipment Cost)

   (1) Minimum assistance       .81
   (2) With assistance         2.06
   (3) Prosthetic training     5.11
   (4) Floor patient           2.20

4.  Relative Value Units

    The minimum total cost for a procedure in Physical Therapy is that for second
    and third modalities, $0.45.  The relative value units for the Gait charges are
    therefore:

    (1) Minimum assistance       .81 ÷ .45 =  2
    (2) With assistance         2.06 ÷ .45 =  5
    (3) Prosthetic training     5.11 ÷ .45 = 11
    (4) Floor patient           2.20 ÷ .45 =  5

**Figure 3.2:** Sample calculation of relative value units for patient charges. (Example: Physical Therapy "gait" charges).

| Procedure | Direct Personnel Cost | Direct Allocated Equip. Cost | Total Direct Cost | RVU | Present RVU |
|---|---|---|---|---|---|
| Modalities | | | | | |
| First Modality | $ 1.04 | $ .34 | $ 1.38 | 3 | 4 |
| Second Modality | .23 | .22 | .45 | 1 | 4 |
| Third Modality | .23 | .22 | .45 | 1 | 4 |
| Vaso Pneumatic | Delete – Charge as Special Procedure | | | | |
| Hydrotherapy | | | | | |
| Hubbard Tank | 9.75 | 1.73 | 11.48 | 26 | 11 |
| Whirlpool – Arm | 4.32 | 1.30 | 5.68 | 12 | 8 |
| Whirlpool H.K.A. + Lower | 5.85 | .97 | 6.85 | 15 | 9 |
| Electrical Stimulation | | | | | |
| A/C, D/C, + Ultrasound | 1.95 | .37 | 2.32 | 5 | |
| Microdyne | 1.11 | .88 | 1.99 | 4 | |
| TENS + EMS | 4.17 | 1.42 | 5.59 | 12 | |
| Fitron | 2.40 | .49 | 2.89 | 6 | 4 |
| Gait | (One charge category broken down into four) | | | | 6 |
| W/Min. Assist. | .73 | .08 | .81 | 2 | |
| W/Assist. | 2.00 | .06 | 2.06 | 5 | |
| Prosthetic Training | 4.96 | .15 | 5.11 | 11 | |
| Floor Patient | 2.16 | .04 | 2.20 | 5 | |
| Group Exercise | Delete – Charge as Therapeutic Exercise Standard Minimal Assist | | | | |
| Home Treatment Instruction | 2.08 | – | 2.08 | 5 | 4 |
| Jobst Meas. B/E, B/K | 2.40 | – | 2.40 | 5 | 4 |
| Jobst Meas. 1 Extrem. | 3.00 | – | 3.00 | 7 | 5 |
| Jobst Meas. 1 Extrem. + TR | 4.20 | – | 4.20 | 9 | 7 |
| Jobst Meas. 2 Extrem. + Trunk | 6.00 | – | 6.00 | 13 | 10 |
| Kinetron | 2.40 | .42 | 2.82 | 6 | 4 |
| Manual Traction | Delete – (none done '80–'81) | | | | |
| Orthotic Fitting | 4.80 | – | 4.80 | 11 | 5 |
| Orthotron | 2.40 | 1.30 | 3.70 | 8 | 4 |
| Patient Burn Care | 4.66 | – | 4.66 | 10 | 3 |
| Patient Eval. (Limited) | 3.06 | – | 3.06 | 7 | 5 |
| Patient Eval. (Regional) | 3.67 | – | 3.67 | 8 | 6 |
| Patient Eval. (General) | 4.90 | – | 4.90 | 11 | 8 |
| Special Procedures | 1.80 | – | 1.80 | 4 | 3 |
| Sweat Test | Delete – Charge as Patient Eval. – General) | | | | |
| Therapeutic Exercise | (Two charge categories broken down into four) | | | | |
| Brief Min. Assist. | 1.60 | .20 | 1.80 | 4 | 4 |
| Brief Max. Assist. | 3.20 | .20 | 3.40 | 8 | 4 |
| Std. Min. Assist. | 1.77 | .30 | 2.07 | 5 | 8 |
| Std. Max. Assist. | 2.95 | .30 | 3.25 | 7 | 8 |
| Tilt Table | 5.25 | .18 | 5.43 | 12 | 7 |
| Traction, Cervical   Combine | | | | | 7 |
| Traction, Pelvic    Combine | | | | | 8 |
| Traction | 4.20 | 5.48 | 9.68 | 21 | |
| Ultrasound | 1.63 | .42 | 2.05 | 5 | 4 |
| Treadmill | Delete – Charge as Gait W/Assist. | | | | |
| Biofeedback | 6.00 | .27 | 6.27 | 14 | 10 |
| Cybex (charge category added) | 4.80 | 9.51 | 14.32 | 32 | 4 |

**Figure 3.3:** Physical therapy direct procedure costs and charge RVUs (Recommended RVUs are rounded off).

| Procedure | Direct Personnel Cost | Direct Allocated Equip. Cost | Total Direct Cost | RVU | Present RVU |
|---|---|---|---|---|---|
| **Activities of Daily Living** | | | | | |
| Brief | $ 2.00 | – | $ 2.00 | 3 | 4 |
| Intermediate | 4.50 | – | 4.50 | 6 | 6 |
| Extended | 6.00 | – | 6.00 | 8 | 9 |
| **Edema Reduction** | | | | | |
| Brief | 1.04 | – | 1.04 | 1 | 4 |
| Intermediate | 1.56 | – | 4.50 | 6 | 6 |
| Extended | 2.86 | – | 6.00 | 8 | 9 |
| **Functional Therapy** | | | | | |
| Brief | .87 | .07 | .94 | 1 | 4 |
| Intermediate | 1.90 | .15 | 2.05 | 3 | 6 |
| Extended | 2.60 | .20 | 2.80 | 4 | 9 |
| **Home Program** | | | | | |
| Brief | 2.40 | – | 2.40 | 3 | 4 |
| Intermediate | 4.80 | – | 4.80 | 7 | 6 |
| Extended | 9.60 | – | 9.60 | 13 | 9 |
| **Evaluation** | | | | | |
| Brief | 2.40 | – | 2.40 | 3 | 4 |
| Intermediate | 4.80 | – | 4.80 | 7 | 6 |
| Extended | 9.60 | – | 9.60 | 13 | 9 |
| **Perceptual Motor Training** | | | | | |
| Brief | .87 | – | .87 | 1 | 4 |
| Intermediate | 1.90 | – | 1.90 | 2 | 6 |
| Extended | 2.60 | – | 2.60 | 4 | 9 |
| **Prosthetic Training** | | | | | |
| Brief | 2.40 | – | 2.40 | 3 | 4 |
| Intermediate | 4.80 | – | 4.80 | 7 | 6 |
| Extended | 9.60 | – | 9.60 | 13 | 9 |
| **Splinting** | | | | | |
| Brief | 2.40 | .30 | 2.70 | 4 | 4 |
| Intermediate | 5.60 | .45 | 5.96 | 8 | 6 |
| Extended | 9.60 | .68 | 10.28 | 14 | 9 |
| **Therapeutic Exercise–Minimal Assistance** | | | | | |
| Brief | .70 | .00 | .70 | 1 | 4 |
| Intermediate | 1.70 | .01 | 1.71 | 2 | 6 |
| Extended | 2.80 | .02 | 2.82 | 4 | 9 |
| **Therapeutic Exercise–Maximal Assistance** | | | | | |
| Brief | 2.40 | .01 | 2.41 | 2 | 4 |
| Intermediate | 5.60 | .04 | 5.64 | 8 | 6 |
| Extended | 9.60 | .06 | 9.66 | 13 | 9 |
| **Work Tolerance** | | | | | |
| Brief | .87 | – | .87 | 1 | 4 |
| Intermediate | 1.90 | – | 1.90 | 2 | 6 |
| Extended | 2.60 | – | 2.60 | 4 | 9 |
| **Group Therapy** | | | | | |
| Brief | $ .96 | – | $ .96 | 1 | 2.5 |
| Intermediate | 1.92 | – | 1.92 | 3 | 3.5 |
| Extended | 3.84 | – | 3.84 | 5 | 5 |
| **Special Procedures** | | | | | |
| Brief | 2.60 | – | 2.60 | 4 | 4 |
| Intermediate | 3.90 | – | 3.90 | 5 | 6 |
| Extended | 5.85 | – | 5.85 | 8 | 9 |
| **Biofeedback** | | | | | |
| Brief | 2.60 | – | 2.60 | 4 | 4 |
| Intermediate | 3.90 | – | 3.90 | 5 | 6 |
| Extended | 5.85 | – | 5.85 | 8 | 9 |

**Figure 3.4:** Occupational therapy direct procedure costs and charge RVUs (Recommended RVUs are founded off).

required for that procedure divided by the time for the procedure with the minimum average time in the service.

The calculation of staff time required to cover peak work load is based on an analysis of the fluctuation and direct patient care work load over the hours of the day. The increase in staff time required, expressed as a percentage of actual direct work load, is illustrated as follows:

1. Determine the average number of patients being treated during each half-hour period of the work day over a two-week sample period.
2. Determine the average and standard deviation of this data set.
3. Percent increase equals the standard deviation divided by the average.

The indirect (non-patient care) staff time required is a constant time allowance. Time for meetings, clinics, patient rounds, reports and general cleaning is included.

Information regarding actual hours worked is obtained from the monthly staff schedules. All sick, vacation, holiday and education time are excluded. A six percent allowance (thirty minutes per day) is made for personal and break time excluding lunch.

## Data Analysis of Patient Scheduling

The analysis of work loads indicated that a 65 percent increase in staffing was necessary in Physical Therapy and 60 percent in Occupational Therapy, just to cover peak periods. Recommendations were made by the management engineer on methods of controlling the extreme fluctuations in work load. After suitable modifications in patient scheduling were implemented, the allowance for peak work load staffing was adjusted to 30 percent in each service.

## Relative Value Units—Implementation and Follow-Up

The implementation of the relative value units (RVU) for patient charges occurred in the spring of 1982. The implementation process involved two steps:

1. Development of total patient charges by the Finance Department. This development required analysis of projected procedure volumes, revenue expectations, and the comparability of the charges with those charges in similar departments. Departmental overhead such as administrative expense and hospital allocated costs were part of the analysis. While the final charges are primarily based on the actual cost, some minor adjustments were made to meet market conditions.
2. Development of a new service sheet and staffing training. The new

service sheet reflects the changes in procedure definitions which were made to more equitably allocate costs based on procedure time and equipment usage.

Although the dollar impact of the new charge system cannot be determined at this point, there are two distinct advantages to the system: Charges are determined according to actual costs; therefore, costs can be more accurately recovered; and charges are more equitably applied to individual procedures; therefore, actual charges to patients are more realistically allocated.

It is planned that the RVU system will be reviewed and revised when major changes occur in methods of performing procedures or staff mix. Routine audits will be conducted every 18–24 months.

## Implementation and Follow-Up of Productivity Monitoring System

The Physical Therapy and Occupational Therapy Services began compiling the productivity monitoring statistics on a monthly basis early in 1982. These statistics provided a comprehensive and objective management tool for setting staffing levels, budgeting for equipment, scheduling meetings, conferences and vacations, and planning new services. Since the implementation of the PM system, the Physical Therapy Service has elected not to fill a registered physical therapy position which became vacant due to staff turnover, and the Occupational Therapy Service upgraded a certified occupational therapy assistant (COTA) position to a registered occupational therapist position, based on information gained from the system.

Whenever the RVU system is revised, as suggested above, or the time allowances used to calculate productivity are adjusted, the worksheets for determining productivity levels will also be revised.

## SUMMARY

The concurrent development of patient charges and productivity monitoring systems provided the Physical and Occupational Therapy Services with comprehensive departmental systems analysis. Through monthly productivity monitoring, the dynamics of the department can be continuously and accurately analyzed. Using the volumes of patient charges as a data base, the productivity monitoring systems provide a link between department staff and equipment utilization and generation of revenue. This provides the department's administrative and management teams with an effective mechanism for planning, organizing, budgeting and controlling services in a confident manner.

# BIBLIOGRAPHY

Kowalski, R. B. and Lippner, L. A. "Development and Implementation of a Relative Charge System for Physical and Occupational Therapy." *Proceedings of a Forum, Productivity Improvements in Physical and Occupational Therapies.* Nashville, Tenn., April 6–7, 1982, 93–106.

Lacourse, E. D. "Application of Statistical Techniques in Staffing and Systems Analysis to Improve Productivity in a Small Department." *Proceedings of the 27th Annual Conference of the American Institute of Industrial Engineers.* St. Louis, Mo., May 18–21, 1976, 178–183.

Oleniacz, S. and Thompson, A. "Self-study of Professional Staffing Requirements." *Proceedings of a Forum, Productivity Improvements in Physical and Occupational Therapies.* Nashville, Tenn., April 6–7, 1982, 163–170.

Picard, G. A. "Development of an Equitable Changing Mechanism for the Department of Physical Medicine Based on a Relative Value System." *Proceedings of a Forum, Productivity Improvements in Physical and Occupational Therapies.* Nashville, Tenn., April 6–7, 75–92.

PHYSICAL THERAPY
PRODUCTIVITY MONITORING MONTHLY WORKSHEET

Period:_____
           (month/year)

I.  Determination of direct work load RVUs required:  From monthly accounting print-
    outs, enter volumes in column B.  Calculate entries in Columns D and E as shown.

| A. Procedure | B. Volume   X<br>(Enter directly<br>From Revenue Report) | RVUs<br>C. Procedure  = | RVUs<br>D. Required<br>(B X C) | PT-RVUs<br>E. Required<br>(Calc. from<br>Column D as<br>indicated) |
|---|---|---|---|---|
| First Modality | _____ | 2.6 | _____ | x 0.25 = _____ |
| Second Modality | _____ | 1.0 | _____ | |
| Third Modality | _____ | 1.0 | _____ | |
| Hydrotherapy | | | | |
| Hubbard Tank | _____ | 20.6 | _____ | |
| Whirlpool – Arm | _____ | 13.0 | _____ | |
| Whirlpool – | | | | |
| K.K.A. + Lower | _____ | 9.6 | _____ | |
| Electrical Stimulation | | | | |
| A/C, D/C + Ultrasound | _____ | 3.1 | _____ | x 0.50 = _____ |
| Microdyne | _____ | 4.3 | _____ | x 0.50 = _____ |
| TENS + EMS | _____ | 6.1 | _____ | x 0.50 = _____ |
| Fitron | _____ | 4.0 | _____ | x 0.50 = _____ |
| Gait | | | | |
| W/Min. Asst. | _____ | 1.8 | _____ | x 0.80 = _____ |
| W/Assist. | _____ | 3.2 | _____ | x 0.50 = _____ |
| Prosthetic Training | _____ | 6.2 | _____ | x 1.00 = _____ |
| Floor Patient | _____ | 2.7 | _____ | x 1.00 = _____ |
| Home Treatment Instruction | _____ | 2.6 | _____ | x 1.00 = _____ |
| Jobst Meas. B/E, B/K | _____ | 4.0 | _____ | x 0.50 = _____ |
| Jobst Meas. 1 Extrem. | _____ | 5.0 | _____ | x 0.50 = _____ |
| Jobst Meas. 1 Extrem. + TR | _____ | 7.0 | _____ | x 0.50 = _____ |
| Jobst Meas. 2 Extrem. | | | | |
| + Trunk | _____ | 10.0 | _____ | x 0.50 = _____ |
| Kinetron | _____ | 4.0 | _____ | x 0.50 = _____ |
| Orthotic Fitting | _____ | 6.0 | _____ | x 1.00 = _____ |
| Orthotron | _____ | 4.0 | _____ | x 0.50 = _____ |
| Patient Burn Care | _____ | 6.0 | _____ | x 0.90 = _____ |
| Patient Eval. (Limited) | _____ | 3.8 | _____ | x 1.00 = _____ |
| Patient Eval. (Regional) | _____ | 4.6 | _____ | x 1.00 = _____ |
| Patient Eval. (General) | _____ | 6.2 | _____ | x 1.00 = _____ |
| Special Procedures | _____ | 3.0 | _____ | x 0.50 = _____ |
| Therapeutic Exercise | | | | |
| Brief Min. Assist. | _____ | 2.0 | _____ | x 1.00 = _____ |
| Brief Max. Assist. | _____ | 4.0 | _____ | x 1.00 = _____ |
| Std. Min. Assist. | _____ | 3.0 | _____ | x 0.67 = _____ |
| Std. Max. Assist. | _____ | 5.0 | _____ | x 0.67 = _____ |
| Tilt Table | _____ | 8.4 | _____ | x 0.50 = _____ |
| Biofeedback | _____ | 10.0 | _____ | x 0.50 = _____ |
| Cybex | _____ | 6.0 | _____ | x 1.00 = _____ |
| TOTAL | | | | |

APPENDIX B

PHYSICAL THERAPY
PRODUCTIVITY MONITORING MONTHLY WORKSHEET

Period: _____
           (month/year)

II.    Enter total of column D........................................ _____

III.   Adjust for peak work load coverage............................ x     1.30
                                                 =  ————————

IV.    Add indirect work load........................................ +  2607.96
                                                 =  ————————

V.     Convert RVUs to hours......................................... x     0.09

          TOTAL HOURS REQUIRED:                          =  ————————

VI.    Calculate actual hours worked:
         Total hours worked*........................................ _____
         Allowance for break time.................................. x     0.94

          TOTAL HOURS WORKED:                           =  ————————

         *(From staff schedules.  Exclude any sick, vacation, holiday or
           outside conference time that occurred this month).

VII.   Calculate productivity:
         Total hours required (from V. above)...................... _____
         Total hours worked (from VI. above)...................... : _____

          PRODUCTIVITY FOR MONTH:                   = _____ %

VIII.  Calculate PT-hours required:
         Enter total of Column E................................... _____
         Adjust for peak work load coverage........................ x _____1.30

                                          =  ————————

         Convert RVUs to hours.................................... x     0.08

         Total PT-hours required for direct work load.............. =  ————————

         Add indirect work load................................... +   153.6

         TOTAL PT-HOURS REQUIRED.................................. =  ————————

         Total hours required (from V. above)..................... _____

         % OF STAFF REQUIRED TO SEE PTs.......................... =

APPENDIX C

PHYSICAL THERAPY
CALCULATION OF FTEs REQUIRED

Period*:_____ to _____
           (month/year)                 (month/year)

*To be calculated based on most recent six months' work load volumes.

   I.   Enter "TOTAL HOURS REQUIRED" from part V of the Productivity
       Worksheet for the six months being considered................    _____

                                                                         +   _____

                                                                        +   _____

                                                                         +   _____

                                                                         +   _____

                                                                         +   _____

                                                                         =   _____

  II.  Adjust for average sick, vacation, holiday, convention,
       and break time............................................... :   .82

                                                                         =   _____

 III.  Convert hours to FTEs........................................ ÷   1040

                                                                         =   _____

---

  IV.  Calculate % of physical therapist required:

       Enter "TOTAL PT-HOURS REQUIRED" from part VIII of the Pro-
       ductivity Worksheets for the six months being considered.....    _____

                                                                         +   _____

                                                                         +   _____

                                                                         +   _____

                                                                         +   _____

                                                                         +   _____
                                                                         =   _____

       TOTAL PT-HOURS REQUIRED:

       Convert hours to FTEs........................................ ÷   852.8

       TOTAL PT-FTEs REQUIRED:                               _____

OCCUPATIONAL THERAPY
PRODUCTIVITY MONITORING MONTHLY WORKSHEET

Period: _____
            (month/year)

I.  Determination of direct work load hours required:  From monthly accounting print-
outs, enter volume in Column B.  Calculate Columns D and E as shown.

| A. Procedure | B. Volume X (Enter directly From Revenue Report) | RVUs C. Procedure = | RVUs D. Required (B X C) | OTR-RVUs E. Required (Calc. from Column D as indicated) |
|---|---|---|---|---|
| **Activities of Daily Living** | | | | |
| Brief | _____ | 2.0 | _____ | |
| Intermediate | _____ | 5.0 | _____ | |
| Extended | _____ | 6.7 | _____ | |
| **Edema Reduction** | | | | |
| Brief | _____ | 1.2 | _____ x 1/2 = _____ | |
| Intermediate | _____ | 1.8 | _____ x 1/2 = _____ | |
| Extended | _____ | 3.4 | _____ x 1/2 = _____ | |
| **Functional Therapy** | | | | |
| Brief | _____ | 1.3 | _____ | |
| Intermediate | _____ | 2.7 | _____ | |
| Extended | _____ | 3.9 | _____ | |
| **Home Program** | | | | |
| Brief | _____ | 1.7 | _____ x 1 = _____ | |
| Intermediate | _____ | 3.3 | _____ x 1 = _____ | |
| Extended | _____ | 6.7 | _____ x 1 = _____ | |
| **Evaluation** | | | | |
| Brief | _____ | 1.7 | _____ x 1 = _____ | |
| Intermediate | _____ | 3.3 | _____ x 1 = _____ | |
| Extended | _____ | 6.7 | _____ x 1 = _____ | |
| **Perceptual Motor Training** | | | | |
| Brief | _____ | 1.2 | _____ | |
| Intermediate | _____ | 2.7 | _____ | |
| Extended | _____ | 3.9 | _____ | |
| **Prosthetic Training** | | | | |
| Brief | _____ | 1.7 | _____ x 1 = _____ | |
| Intermediate | _____ | 3.3 | _____ x 1 = _____ | |
| Extended | _____ | 6.7 | _____ x 1 = _____ | |
| **Splinting** | | | | |
| Brief | _____ | 1.7 | _____ x 1 = _____ | |
| Intermediate | _____ | 3.9 | _____ x 1 = _____ | |
| Extended | _____ | 6.7 | _____ x 1 = _____ | |
| **Therapeutic Exercise- Minimal Assistance** | | | | |
| Brief | _____ | 1.1 | _____ x 1/2 = _____ | |
| Intermediate | _____ | 2.4 | _____ x 1/2 = _____ | |
| Extended | _____ | 4.1 | _____ x 1/2 = _____ | |
| **Therapeutic Exercise- Maximal Assistance** | | | | |
| Brief | _____ | 1.7 | _____ x 1/2 = _____ | |
| Intermediate | _____ | 3.9 | _____ x 1/2 = _____ | |
| Extended | _____ | 6.7 | _____ x 1/2 = _____ | |

APPENDIX D (Cont.)

## OCCUPATIONAL THERAPY
## PRODUCTIVITY MONITORING MONTHLY WORKSHEET

Period: _____
         (month/year)

I.  Determination of direct work load hours required:  From monthly acounting print-
    outs, enter volumes in column B.  Calculate Columns D and E as shown.

| A. Procedure | B. Volume X (Enter directly From Revenue Report) | RVUs C. Procedure = | RVUs D. Required (B X C) | OTR-RVUs E. Required (Calc. from Column D as indicated) |
|---|---|---|---|---|
| Work Tolerance | | | | |
| Brief | _____ | 1.2 | _____ x 1 = | _____ |
| Intermediate | _____ | 2.7 | _____ x 1 = | _____ |
| Extended | _____ | 3.9 | _____ x 1 = | _____ |
| Group Therapy | | | | |
| Brief | _____ | 1.0 | _____ x 1 = | _____ |
| Intermediate | _____ | 1.9 | _____ x 1 = | _____ |
| Extended | _____ | 3.7 | _____ x 1 = | _____ |
| Special Procedures | | | | |
| Brief | _____ | 2.2 | _____ x 1/2 = | _____ |
| Intermediate | _____ | 3.3 | _____ x 1/2 = | _____ |
| Extended | _____ | 5.0 | _____ x 1/2 = | _____ |
| Biofeedback | | | | |
| Brief | _____ | 2.2 | _____ x 1/2 = | _____ |
| Intermediate | _____ | 3.3 | _____ x 1/2 = | _____ |
| Extended | _____ | 5.0 | _____ x 1/2 = | _____ |
| TOTAL | | | | |

APPENDIX E

OCCUPATIONAL THERAPY
PRODUCTIVITY MONITORING MONTHLY WORKSHEET

Period: _____
          (month/year)

II.  Enter total of column D........................................ _____

III.  Adjust for peak work load coverage........................... x     1.30
                                               = _____

IV.  Add indirect work load....................................... +    825.56
                                               = _____

V.  Convert RVUs to hours........................................ x     0.15
                                               = _____

    TOTAL HOURS REQUIRED:

VI.  Calculate actual hours worked
    Total hours worked*.........................................
    Allowance for break time.................................... x     0.94
                                           

    TOTAL HOURS WORKED

    *(From staff schedules.  Exclude any sick, vacation, holiday or
    outside conference time that occurred this month.)

VII.  Calculate productivity:
    Total hours required (from V. above).........................  _____
    Total hours worked (from VI. above).......................... :  _____

    PRODUCTIVITY FOR MONTH:                  = _____ %

VIII.  Calculate OTR-hours required:
    Enter total of Column E.....................................
    Adjust for peak work load coverage.......................... x  _____1.30
                                           = _____

    Convert RVUs to hours....................................... x  _____0.15
                                           = _____

    Total OTR-hours required for direct work load..............

    Add indirect work load...................................... +    96.9
                                           = _____

    TOTAL OTR-HOURS REQUIRED...................................

    Total hours required (from V. above).......................  _____
                                           = _____

    % OF STAFF REQUIRED TO BE OTRs.............................

59

APPENDIX F

OCCUPATIONAL THERAPY
CALCULATION OF FTEs REQUIRED

Period\*_____ to _____
　　　　　　(month/year)　　　　　　　　　　(month/year)

\*To be calculated based on most recent six months' work load volumes.

  I.   Enter "TOTAL HOURS REQUIRED" from part V of the Productivity
      Worksheet for the six months being considered................  _____

                                                                 +  _____

                                                                 +  _____

                                                                 +  _____

                                                                 +  _____

                                                                 +  _____

                                                                 =  ==========

  II.  Adjust for average sick, vacation, holiday, convention,
      and break time........................................... ÷     .82

 III.  Convert hours to FTEs...................................... =   1040
                                                                           ==========

---

  IV.  Calculate % of occupational therapist requred:

      Enter "TOTAL OT-HOURS REQUIRED" from part VIII of the Pro-
      ductivity Worksheets for the six months being considered...  _____

                                                                   +  _____

                                                                 +  _____

                                                                 +  _____

                                                                 +  _____

                                                                 +  _____

                TOTAL OT-HOURS REQUIRED           +  ==========

      Convert hours to FTEs...................................... ÷   852.8

                TOTAL OT-FTEs REQUIRED:               ==========

*Melva Diamante,* MBA

# 4   Performance Review in Rehabilitation Service

## INTRODUCTION

Human resources constitute a major component of health care institutions and the management of this resource is undoubtedly a significant factor in the delivery of patient care. Today, management in the health care environment is continually being challenged by the escalating cost of operation, demand for quality patient care, governmental requirements, the changing nature of the workforce, and decreasing productivity. The health care organization which will survive is the one in which managers have mastered the skills and techniques of motivating employees to perform their roles more productively. One of the initial steps toward enhancing performance is the ongoing appraisal of the employee's work.

Performance appraisal or review refers to the process of evaluating an employee's work efforts, output, or results based upon specific standards and expectations set for the job. Performance appraisal includes the ongoing process of formal and informal, specific and general, feedback with which supervisors provide employees and the periodic documentation of the appraisal followed by an evaluation discussion.

One concern that is being raised by my colleagues in the Association of Hospital Personnel Administrators is that many health care institutions still use the same performance appraisal form for all levels and categories of employees. Many institutions which have developed performance review systems use one type of performance review instrument regardless of whether an employee is working in an office, a laboratory, or is directly involved with delivery of patient care.

In some institutions, services such as Rehabilitation, Nursing, and others are permitted to develop and use their own performance review forms if they are consistent with the institution's performance review philosophy. In many others, however, this option of designing an appraisal form to meet the unique needs of a specific service does not exist.

For those managers who have to conduct performance reviews within an established and structured system, this article presents an

approach to planning the evaluation process, supplementing the standard review form, documenting the performance review, and conducting the performance evaluation interview with the employee. Moreover,
it provides guidelines for conducting management and staff performance reviews applicable to a rehabilitation service setting. This article
raises issues and provides guidelines for those who are evaluating
current or proposed performance review systems for rehabilitation
services.

## WHY HAVE PERFORMANCE REVIEWS?

Evaluation, in general, is not a new concept in rehabilitation services; it
is a major concern of rehabilitation professionals whose primary objective is the delivery of quality patient care. Rehabilitation services are
acutely aware of the need for the continuous evaluation of all phases of
their operation, from their organization, utilization and quality of services, to the arrangements made for transfer, discharge, and follow-up
of patients. Performance review is an essential component of this overall
assessment process which every rehabilitation unit is required to conduct by the government and the therapists' professional affiliations.

Evaluation and development of staff are requirements in any quality
assurance program as well as in efforts of a hospital to gain accreditation
from the Joint Commission on Accreditation of Hospitals (JCAH). Dale
and McDonald indicate that rehabilitation facilities need staff evaluation
for accreditation by the Commission on Accreditation of Rehabilitation
Facilities (CARF). The Personnel section of the Standard Manual for
Rehabilitation Facilities (CARF, 1981) stipulates that "a job performance
evaluation shall be conducted for each staff member on a regular basis
by the immediate supervisor, and the results shall be documented,
reviewed with the staff person, and then included in the personnel
file."[1]

Performance appraisal is not only an evaluative instrument, but also
a motivational and developmental tool of management. Performance
review has been used as a basis for decisions concerning salary increases, promotions, and other similar personnel actions. Beyond this
evaluative role, the performance review process opens up lines of
communication between supervisor and employee. Both are provided
with the opportunity to review and clarify the employee's responsibilities, the supervisor's expectations, and the performance standards.
When performance appraisals are conducted properly, they help managers motivate, train, and develop employees and reinforce or modify
their behavior.

As Levinson points out, the significant functions of performance evaluations are to:

- measure and judge performance
- relate individual performance to individual goals
- clarify both the job to be done and the expectations
- foster the compliance and growth of subordinate
- enhance communication between supervisor and subordinate
- serve as a basis for judgments about salary and promotions, and
- stimulate the subordinate's motivation and serve as a device for organizational control and utilization.[2]

## PERFORMANCE REVIEW PROCESS

In order to maximize favorable results the performance review process should include the following steps: (1) description of the employee's duties and responsibilities, (2) setting goals, (3) developing performance standards, and (4) evaluation of performance and discussion of the evaluation with the employee (see Figure 4.1). The relationship of these steps to each other is very much like those steps in a staircase. It is both supportive and progressive. The first step supports the second and the first two steps support the third and so on. The final step in the process, performance evaluation can only truly exist when the three prior steps have been successfully accomplished.

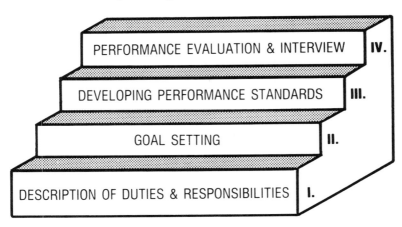

PERFORMANCE EVALUATION & INTERVIEW IV.

DEVELOPING PERFORMANCE STANDARDS III.

GOAL SETTING II.

DESCRIPTION OF DUTIES & RESPONSIBILITIES I.

**Figure 4.1:** Performance Review Process

## Description of Duties and Responsibilities

As a starting point, a job description should be written which includes, at the very least, the employee's duties, responsibilities, accountabilities and knowledge and skill requirements. The employee's participation in the preparation or revision of the job description must be encouraged as it creates a sense of ownership which enhances the employee's understanding of what he or she is expected to do and contributes to the employee's concurrence and acceptance of responsibilities. Job description writing clarifies objectives of the position and allows both the supervisor and the employee to highlight critical aspects of the job. As Henderson says, one of the best, possibly the only, approach available to management for achieving employee awareness, understanding, and acceptance of goals is to involve employees as much as possible in the planning, operation, and control of workplace activities.[3]

Since responsibilities do change over time, the supervisor and employee are expected to review and update the job description periodically or whenever major changes in responsibilities or duties occur. The significance of a change in responsibility will be determined by its impact on the overall objectives of the job. In preparing or revising the job description, the supervisor should consult the organization's human resources (or personnel) staff.

## Goal Setting

The next step in the performance review process is goal setting. The employee's job description and past work performance are the bases for developing future goals. In general, there are three types of goals. One type is directed at correcting a specific problem. The second type of goal is intended to improve past performance or to improve the existing operation. The assumption here is that the current levels of performance or operation are acceptable but efforts will be made to progress to higher levels. The third type of goal is aimed at maintaining current levels of performance or operation. The assumption here is that the existing levels of performance are more than acceptable or are excellent and the goal is to maintain the status quo.

Performance improves when goal setting takes into consideration: (1) employee involvement in the process, (2) establishing specific goals, (3) including specific action steps to be taken, and (4) establishing goals that are challenging.

> Setting effective goals is important for several reasons. Often, when an employee's performance is inadequate it is not because he or she does not want to do better, but because he or she either thinks he is doing what is expected, or does not know what is expected. (Sometimes, in

fact, just showing an employee how he is actually performing relative to his standard may be enough to bring his performance back into line.) Similarly, employees have to first understand what is expected of them before consequences like pay can motivate the desired behavior.[4]

The supervisor's role is especially critical in ensuring that the employee does not set unrealistic or irrelevant goals. Aiming too high will result in frustration when the employee fails to realize the target. On the other hand, an employee may set goals that are easily attainable knowing that they will be bases for performance evaluation. Setting the goals too low is not only counter-productive but also stifles an individual's growth and development. Locke has conducted a number of studies concerning the role of goal setting in improving work performance. Based on his findings, Locke concludes that (1) hard goals result in higher levels of performance than do easy goals and (2) that specific hard goals result in a higher level of performance than do no goals or a generalized goal of "do your best."[5]

Prior to meeting with the supervisor, an employee should be asked to establish goals and identify action steps to be taken for a specific period of time. Action steps include various key activities that have to be performed in order to achieve the goals. Goals can be both short and long term. The significance of the employee's involvement in goal setting is summarized by Edward Lawler as follows:

> People become "ego involved" in decisions in which they have had influence. The decisions become their decisions and they develop expectancies to the effect that when decisions are successfully implemented they will experience such intrinsic rewards as feelings of confidence and self-esteem. Because of this they work to implement this decision even though no extrinsic rewards are involved.[6]

After the employee has set his or her goals, the supervisor and employee will discuss them, prioritize these goals and review the action steps. These action steps should be specific and should include resource requirements (financial, equipment, training, staffing, supervisory support, etc.). In addition, the goal statement has to indicate the timeframe within which the activities will be performed or completed. Review checkpoints will be designated and will specify points in time for review of the employee's progress.

In setting goals one has to refer to each of the functional areas in the employee's job description. For instance, in the case of a management employee, the functional areas may include planning, organizing, staffing, directing, activating, coordinating, and controlling. The manner in which a management employee performs these functions would depend upon the organizational structure. Regardless of organizational differences the supervisor and the employee will have to go through the same goal setting process.

Figure 4.2 is an illustration of how goals could be established for management employees in a rehabilitation service. Goals are listed for two functional areas, i.e., staffing and controlling.

In the illustration, the goals listed for the staffing role of the employee indicate an attempt to correct problems in the quality of therapists hired and an apparently high turnover rate. For the controlling function, the stated goals are aimed at (1) improving existing methods of record keeping and (2) maintaining existing levels of performance specifically in complying with government regulations. The action steps are listed for each goal. The statement of goals should also include time tables for each action step. In addition resource requirements to accomplish these goals should be indicated. For example, as part of the action step the employee may need the assistance of peers or staff therapists or money to be budgeted in order to expand internship programs.

Figure 4.3 illustrates how goals and action steps could be developed for a rehabilitation service staff. The example indicates goals and specific activities for three functional areas. These functional areas are extracted from the staff's job description.

## Developing Performance Standards

After goals and action steps are developed, the supervisor and the employee will discuss the expected results and performance standards for each of these goals. Furthermore, performance standards will be established for all key performance criteria. These criteria consist of factors which are required in order to perform the job successfully. In organizations which have formal performance review systems, the performance criteria are listed in the appraisal form. It is common for these forms to include such criteria as quality and quantity of work, timeliness, the employee's relationship with co-workers, attendance, punctuality, cooperation with others, initiative, and other similar dimensions.

These criteria or dimensions differ from position to position depending upon the positions' objectives, level, complexity, and skill and knowledge requirements.

As indicated earlier in this article, use of standard performance review forms for all types and levels of employees can be a source of concern. This is because supervisors are forced to evaluate employees using irrelevant criteria and at the same time overlook key dimensions of the employee's job. However, a supervisor can still effectively evaluate an employee within the constraints of the institutional format. The

| Functional Areas | Goals | Action Steps |
|---|---|---|
| 1. Staffing | 1. Hire more qualified therapists as vacancies occur | 1. Expand internship program by involving participation of other schools. |
| | | 2. Identify specific key or critical job requirements and communicate them to the Personnel Department as recruitment and selection guides. |
| | | 3. Receive training in interviewing selection techniques. |
| | 2. Reduce turnover by 50% | 1. Open lines of communication with staff and other supervisors in the service. Meet two times a month to discuss problems, progress of work, etc. |
| | | 2. Review periodically work progress and problems with staff. |
| | | 3. Identify and respond to motivational needs of staff. Conduct one-to-one sessions with staff every two months. |
| 2. Controlling | 1. Establish more efficient methods for reviewing documentation of patient care | 1. Investigate feasibility of using peer review. |
| | | 2. Review documentation standards/procedures. Prepare a proposal to improve methods. |
| | 2. Maintain compliance with governmental regulations and Quality Assurance Program requirements | 1. Assess treatment methods, quality and appropriateness of care provided (e.g. every six months). |
| | | 2. Ascertain accurate and complete documentation of treatment and progress of patients are maintained. |
| | | 3. Maintain continuing update of policy and procedure manual. |

**Figure 4.2:** Sample of goal statement for a management employee.

supervisor and the employee should develop a list of criteria. This will include all the relevant criteria which are contained in the existing performance appraisal form and other additional dimensions which are required in order to meet the objectives of the job. Each of these criteria has to be clearly defined and agreed upon by both the supervisor and employee.

Performance criteria for management employees are expected to be different from those of the rest of the staff. Some examples of performance criteria for management employees in a rehabilitation service are as follows:

**Planning.** Develops realistic plans and involves appropriate staff in the planning process; establishes an effective course of action for self and unit in order to establish goals and objectives.

**Organization.** Utilizes available resources in order to maximize effectiveness of the rehabilitation service. Establishes the organizational

| Functional Areas | Goals | Action Steps |
|---|---|---|
| 1. Treatment Plan Development | 1. Develop treatment program for newly opened oncology ward | 1. Visit 2 other facilities with rehabilitation programs for oncology patients. |
| | | 2. Attend at least, two workshops on oncology patients and rehabilitation related programs, i.e., death and dying, etc. |
| | | 3. Write an O.T. treatment protocol for oncology patients. |
| 2. Clinical Student Supervision | 1. Act as preceptor for one of the interns | 1. Attend preceptor training seminar. |
| | | 2. Write a preceptor's teaching plan for assigned intern. |
| | | 3. Conduct and report to Chief Therapist the evaluation of intern. |
| 3. Patient Evaluation | 1. Apply S.O.A.P.ier (Subjective-Objective-Assessment-Plan imple-tation and program evaluation/revision format) | 1. Attend workshop on S.O.A.P. implementation and program evaluation/revision format. |
| | | 2. Rewrite and submit to Chief Therapist reports of previous patients using the S.O.A.P. implementation and program evaluation/revision format. |

**Figure 4.3:** Sample of goal statement for staff.

structure, i.e., relationships between staff, work and physical resources. Integrates the various activities and services needed to deliver total patient care. Develops written policies and procedures for efficiency of operation and quality patient care.

**Interpersonal Relationship.** Understands human behavior and uses that in guiding and directing efforts of others to realize the unit's objectives; firm and fair in dealing with staff and associates, follows established personnel policies and procedures.

**Controlling.** Develops a program for periodic assessment of quality and appropriateness of care, establishes quality control including performance against budgets. Coordinates efforts with medical staff and other medical personnel in evaluating the rehabilitation programs/services.

**Communication.** Organizes ideas and expresses them effectively, both verbally and in writing; maintains open lines of communication with peers, supervisors, staff, and other medical professionals who are involved in providing care to the unit's patients.

**Decision Making.** Recognizes problems and takes appropriate corrective action. Analyzes the unit's needs, arrives at timely and appropriate course of action.

**Staff Development.** Provides employees with tools necessary for them to realize expected levels of performance on the job; develops subordinates by delegating to them and by encouraging them to pursue training.

For a staff therapist some suggested criteria are:

**Knowledge.** Develops effective treatment plans; keep up-to-date with developments in treatment techniques and demonstrates this knowledge in decisions concerning patient treatment.

**Organization.** Integrates responsibilities independently; effectively uses resources, personnel, and equipment to achieve job objectives.

**Problem Solving.** Analyzes problems affecting work, considers alternatives and chooses appropriate courses of action. Uses judgment in responding to contingency; creative and resourceful in dealing with contingencies.

**Communication.** Effectively conveys information to supervisor, co-worker, patients, and other individuals, whose activities affect the employee's work and the work objectives. Maintains complete and accurate records of patient's prognosis, referral, treatment and progress.

**Relationship with Co-Workers.** Works with others, individually and in groups. Provides assistance to co-workers when help is solicited; contributes to team effort resulting in better patient care. Resolves conflicts which interfere with achievement of the job objectives.

**Dependability.** Seeks and assumes responsibility; carries out responsibility in a thorough and timely manner.

**Work Habits.** Complies with established administrative and clinical policies and procedures. Implements treatment plans effectively. Works with treatment teams to determine most appropriate treatment approach for patient. Meets attendance and punctuality regulations.

**Self-Development.** Participates in in-house training or educational activities. Participates in continuing education and other available professional/developmental opportunities and shares knowledge with co-workers.

The supervisor and employee must establish clearly defined performance standards for each of the criteria and goals. While performance criteria are broad or general statements of job requirements, performance standards include specific and if possible, quantifiable statements of expectation. Standards should be:

- results oriented
- objective
- challenging
- useful, and
- realistic.

A performance standard emphasizes results. As Rowland points out, it is a written statement of conditions that will exist when a job is being well done:[7]

> . . . Standards of performance say how well, rather than what. They spell out the targets or expectations of an individual and the supervisor in connection with a given job. Through analysis of each major segment, a series of standards or specific goals for performance is developed. These can be used later to judge whether or not the total job is being performed satisfactorily. Meanwhile, they represent an agreement on the goals of the job holder.[8]

Standards are objective when they are specific and results-oriented. While it is not possible to quantify all performance standards, there are ways of establishing some measurable indices. Aside from establishing absolute numbers or percentage requirements, standards could include frequency of occurrences or specific time frames within which activities should be completed or specific dollar-limits.

Standards should also be challenging and aimed at stretching the individual's ability or levels of performance. For instance, if the goal in the previous review period was to complete initial evaluation reports within seven days seventy percent of the time, the standard for the current review could be raised to completion of initial evaluation within five days eighty percent of the time.

Employees will be motivated to meet or even exceed the standards when they are perceived to be useful both for the organization and the employee. When the employee perceives a connection between his or her own personal goals and the standards, the latter has a motivational effect on the employee. A performance standard is also effective when it is perceived as contributing toward the unit's objective. The employee will develop a sense of purpose in realizing the expected results. A performance standard is realistic when it is achievable. Both the supervisor and the employee must have an understanding and agreement on what constitutes attainable standards or expectations.

The supervisor will ensure that the standards are clearly defined and that the employee understands them. The supervisor and the employee must agree on what constitutes acceptable, unacceptable or outstanding performance. Appraisal systems provide for a variety of scales of performance. Whatever method is used, standards must be applied consistently. In setting or changing standards the supervisor might have to allow flexibility in order to meet variations in resource allocations and changing conditions.

## Performance Evaluation and Interview

Performance reviews do not consist only of the periodic and formal documentation of the employee's job performance; they also include an ongoing process of discussion between supervisor and employee concerning the latter's work progress. This continuing dialogue is especially necessary when the goals and activities are tied to specific time tables. The purpose of these ongoing discussions is to:

- review the progress of the employee's work or projects
- identify problems, if any
- resolve problems
- reassure the employee of the supervisor's interest in and support of the employee's work, and
- give the employee feedback which will eliminate suprises when the formal documented performance review takes place.

The final step in the performance review process includes documenting the performance evaluation and discussing it with the employee. This final step requires thoughtful preparation for the evaluation, completion of the performance appraisal form or documentation of the evaluation, and conducting the evaluation interview.

*Preparation for Evaluation Interview.* Prior to conducting the performance interview, a great deal of preparation and planning takes place. The supervisor reviews the goals set for the job and determines the goals which were achieved and those not achieved. The supervisor will review the critical job criteria and the performance standards and compare them with actual results. Accomplishments and shortfalls will also be identified. Since the supervisor cannot rely solely upon memory, he or she must consult the list of observations that were gathered throughout the review period. This list will include observations documented in a log indicating types of incidents, dates of occurrence, probable causes of problem situations, and action in response to each problem. Poor performance and anything that exceeds average performance should be noted in this log. With these observations, patterns of behavior which affect success or failure on the job must be identified. The supervisor should consult other people who are in a position to evaluate some aspects of the employee's performance. For instance, if staff are rotated among different areas of the service and they work under different unit supervisors or medical professionals, their assessment of the employee's performance could be solicited and considered for the evaluation process. Results of audit programs which review patient charts completed by employees are important sources of information for the employee's evaluation.

Employee involvement should be invited during the preparation period. Prior to the discussion the employee may be asked to review his or her performance by thinking of the goals discussed earlier during the review period, the performance criteria and standards, and actual results.

*Documenting Performance Appraisal.* In documenting the evaluation, the employee's performance must be compared with the standards defined at the beginning of the review period. The supervisor will provide specific examples both for good as well as poor performance. It is important to be objective in the evaluation process. Subjectivity is a common error which plagues the appraisal system. While this problem may be due to the supervisor's biases, it can also result from the shortcomings of the system itself. A performance review tool which requires the supervisor to rate personality traits, for example, is bound to generate highly subjective evaluations.

There are appraisal systems which do not provide an objective basis for evaluation, or do not clearly define the evaluation criteria or the performance standards. In these cases, evaluation becomes highly subjective. Some organizations do not provide supervisors with training in evaluation techniques. A supervisor should be given training on conducting a performance review before evaluating employees.

With some supervisors, bias may be due to preconceived notions about the employees' ethnic group, age, or sex. One study showed that high performing females tend to be rated significantly higher than high performing males. Low performing blacks tend to be rated significantly higher than low performing whites.[9] There are others who are influenced by the halo effect. This is a tendency to rate a person consistently according to the supervisor's general impression about the person. For instance, if the supervisor is impressed with the employee's educational background, he or she gives the employee a high performance rating. If the supervisor believes that the employee is a good person, most of this employee's rating will be high. If he or she believes that the employee is a poor performer, the supervisor will find it difficult to find any good point in favor of this employee.[10]

Another common mistake is what DuBrin calls "constant error," which is a tendency among supervisors to use only one portion of the scale in rating employees.[11] Some evaluators find it difficult and uncomfortable to confront employees with low ratings and find an easy way out by being lenient in rating employees in the middle of the scale. A marginal performer who is rated by the lenient supervisor thinks that he or she is doing well and there is no reason to correct or change work habits. On the other hand, a good performer is demotivated because he or she is rated equally as a marginal performer. Other supervisors take the opposite extreme and maintain a reputation in the organization as "tough boss to work for." An unreasonably strict evaluator generates frustration among employees so the appraisal becomes a tool for demotivating employees. This is especially true when employees do not understand why excellence in performance is not recognized and rewarded by the review process.

*Conducting the Performance Evaluation and Interview.* Although it is an easy and pleasant task to provide positive feedback to an employee, giving negative comments is challenging and may create a problem for the supervisor. The employee knows that the performance appraisal will affect his or her job security, promotional opportunity, and possibly, pay increase. The supervisor's success in conducting the evaluation interview is important as it could lead to good working relations between the supervisor and the employee, open up lines of communication between them and enhance employee motivation.

The interview is of a confidential and personal nature. Therefore, the supervisor must conduct the discussion in a private, quiet office, away from telephone and people distractions.

A brief, but thoughtful introduction to the evaluation interview may make the difference between a successful or unsuccessful review.[12] The employee could be made comfortable by creating a cordial atmosphere. The discussion could be started with "small talk," something unrelated to the review session. Then the purpose of the interview should be stated. The supervisor must encourage a dialogue. As a springboard for discussion, the employee and supervisor may compare their evaluations of the employee's performance. Differences in their evaluation ought to be discussed and the employee should be made to understand that the supervisor's evaluation could change based upon new information resulting from the dialogue. Positive feedback should be given by showing examples and discussing the factors which may have contributed to successful results. This helps reinforce preferred behavior and work habits.

In providing negative feedback the supervisor should also discuss specific results and why results are what they are, without reference to personalities, traits, or attitudes.

> In order for criticism to be constructive, it must be specific and must provide the employee with all the information needed for a good performance. Don't say "You haven't got the right attitude" or say "You should be more careful." Tell subordinates the details which have been left undone.
>
> Criticisms which can be interpreted as an attack not only fail to clear up mistakes, but often worsen performance as well. People criticized in this way rarely absorb what you tell them. Every person needs to keep a high self-opinion; by attacking self image, you only succeed in producing hostility and damaging feelings. Tell subordinates what is wrong with their work, not themselves.[13]

The employee's participation is crucial as it may help uncover factors or conditions beyond the employee's control which may have caused the problem. The supervisor must encourage an open discussion and be receptive to suggestions made by the employee.

The objectives of the interview are to review performance together, congratulate the employee for his or her accomplishments, identify shortcomings and the reasons for them, develop a plan for addressing these deficiencies or problems, review developmental and training tools, and establish goals for the next review period. The participation of the employee is necessary not only in identifying shortcomings but also in developing an action plan to respond to these deficiencies. This involvement gives the employee a sense of ownership for the action plan and its implementation.

The interview may be ended when both supervisor and employee are in agreement that the discussion achieved the purpose stated at the beginning of the session and when the supervisor believes that the employee has been given full opportunity to share his or her thoughts about the performance evaluation. A successful interview session is one which ends with the employee developing a sense of pride for his or her accomplishments, understanding the value of maintaining performance at a high level and at the same time, recognizing the importance of improving problem areas which were identified in the discussion.

The employee's participation in the entire performance review process is of utmost importance. This involvement contributes to making performance evaluation an effective instrument for management.

## SUMMARY

This article presented guidelines for rehabilitation services managers on how to plan and conduct performance reviews. The purpose here was twofold:

1. to provide an approach to planning and conducting a performance evaluation for those who must work within the constraints of an established performance review system. The focus is to maximize the utilization of the existing performance evaluation tool.
2. to raise issues and provide guidance in the design and development of a performance evaluation system.

Performance review was described as an instrument of management which should be used to evaluate as well as motivate and develop employees. Furthermore, it was seen as a mechanism necessary for compliance with various government and regulatory agency requirements.

The process of performance review was characterized as having four supportive and progressive steps. These included:

1. description of the employee's duties and responsibilities
2. setting goals for the employee
3. development of performance standards
4. evaluation of performance and discussion of the evaluation with the employee.

Joint participation of the supervisor and employee was emphasized as a crucial element of all the steps in the process.

## NOTES

1. B. Dale and A. A. McDonald, Sr., "Towards a Comprehensive Philosophy of Personnel Performance Appraisal in Rehabilitation Facilities," *Journal of Rehabilitation Administration*, May 1982, 80.

2. H. Levison, "Management by Whose Objectives," *Howard Business Review*, July–August, 1970, 126. See also A. C. Bennett, *Improving Management Performance in Health Care Institutions, A Total System Approach* (Ill.: American Hospital Association, 1978).

3. R. I. Henderson, *Performance Appraisal: Theory to Practice* (Reston, Va.: Reston Publishing Co., Inc., 1980), 87.

4. G. Dessler, *Human Behavior—Improving Productivity at Work* (Reston, Va.: Reston Publishing Co., Inc., 1980), 169.

5. E. Locke, N. Cartledge, and C. S. Kerr, "Studies of the Relationship between Satisfaction, Goal Setting, and Performance," *Organizational Behavior and Human Behavior*, 1970, 135–158.

6. Dessler, *Human Behavior*, 175.

7. V. K. Rowland, *Managerial Performance Standards* (New York: American Management Association, 1960), 35–36.

8. Ibid.

9. W. J. Bigoness, "Effects of Applicant's Sex, Race, and Performance on Employer's Performance Ratings: Some Additional Findings," *Journal of Applied Psychology*, February 1976, 84.

10. R. W. Eckles, R. L. Carmichael, and B. R. Sarchet, *Supervisory Management* (New York: John Wiley & Sons, Inc., 1981), 384.

11. A. J. DuBrin, *Personnel and Human Resource Management* (New York: D. Van Nostrand Co., 1981), 132.

12. Henderson, *Performance Appraisal*, 119.

13. G. G. Alpander, "Training First-Line Supervisors to Criticize Constructively," *Personnel Journal*, March 1980, 220.

*Jan Harrington,* RPT

# 5 Assessing Philosophies of Treatment

## INTRODUCTION

The treatment philosophy is the framework out of which therapists approach both their work and individual patients. It is the basic underlying interaction that occurs between the health professional and the patient. Just as one's philosophy of life affects one's values and beliefs, and determines one's lifestyle, so the philosophy of treatment affects therapists' approach to patients, the roles therapists assume, and the results of the therapy.

In order for the rehabilitative professionals to better understand themselves and what they have to offer, they must find ways to identify, define, and assess the basic treatment philosophies. Assessment of philosophies entails more than comparing treatment methods (e.g., comparing therapeutic exercise versus physical agent), and it is more than defining an approach (e.g., the Bobath "approach" to treatment). An analogy would be that the method or approach is the tool, while the philosophy of treatment is the workshop.

## PURPOSE

The purpose of this paper is to encourage therapy administrators in assisting the staff to identify, assess and critically appraise their philosophies of treatment. Components of treatment philosophies will be discussed, and the assessment process will be explained. Following this, the author will present a framework for identifying two treatment philosophies within a home health agency. A study will then be presented which illustrates one way in which treatment philosophies may be researched. Hopefully, the text as well as the research study will stimulate new thoughts regarding the relationships among treatment philosophies, treatment settings and treatment outcomes.

## IDENTIFYING TREATMENT PHILOSOPHIES

Webster defines philosophy as: "The logical analysis of the principles underlying conduct, thought and knowledge; a particular system of principles for the conduct of life." Applying this definition to the therapists' professional lives involves three basic steps: first, therapists must identify a concept of self in the professional role. What are the therapists' values, attitudes and beliefs about ease and effectiveness in dealing with patients (e.g., cultural differences; dealing with a patient with a terminal diagnosis). Second, therapists must identify their professional *modus operandi*. Into which professional practices do their values, attitudes and beliefs lead them? In what form of interaction with patients are they most comfortable and most effective? Third, therapists must identify the external factors which may require a modification of their preferred *modus operandi*. Does the patient have an effective support system? Are there language barriers to consider? What are the patient's expectations and motivations? How do these factors affect the therapists' selection process for modifying their interaction?

Treatment philosophy is the basic pattern of interaction underlying all that is done in relationship to patients. It is the framework within which the professional is most at ease, and consequently is most effective with patients. There are many implications when considering treatment philosophies and their relative effectiveness. As areas of professional involvement become more complex, and as therapists become more specialized, identifying treatment philosophies and assessing the effectiveness of those philosophies become increasingly important.

## ASSESSMENT PROCESS

To assess is "to determine the relative value, significance, or importance of," according to Webster. In assessing philosophies of treatment, therapists must have a scientific mind-set that is willing to risk disclosure and is open to revision. They must be able to think through all of the factors that may differentially affect what they do with what they believe. There are external factors to consider, both patient-related and environmental. There are the effects of professional training and experiences, or limitations of job opportunities. There are personal factors for each therapist, such as degrees of assertiveness and personal/ professional goals. All of these must be considered when determining the importance of one's philosophy.

To identify a philosophy of treatment is basic to one's professional identity. To assess that philosophy and determine its relative importance is basic to one's professional integrity. To critically appraise one's philosophy is to "come of age" as professionals in a chosen field.

## CRITICAL APPRAISAL

Critically appraising the therapists' philosophies of treatment consists of determining the relative effectiveness of their philosophies in terms of treatment outcomes. What difference does one's philosophy make in terms of objectively measured treatment effectiveness? Does positive subjective information from the patients regarding their perceptions of treatment correlate with what the professional may describe as "effective" treatment? By comparing philosophies of a staff of therapists, the therapy administrator may discover that one philosophy is more effective in one setting than in another. Perhaps the administrator then can develop ways to match professionals with job opportunities to decrease burn-out and staff turn-over rates. Perhaps philosophies of treatment exist which prove to be effective in terms of outcome regardless of setting.

## IDENTIFYING A PHILOSOPHICAL FRAMEWORK

There are several factors to consider when attempting to identify and compare philosophies of treatment. Some of these factors are the philosophy and goals of the facility or agency; the treatment setting; the individual philosophies and goals of the staff, and whether or not these provide a basis for comparison; the cost of services and factors affecting those costs and generation of revenue.

In the non-profit health agency where the study to be presented was performed, the author was requested by administration to prove the effectiveness of a particular philosophy of treatment. The initial effect of that philosophy was a decrease in revenue due to a decrease in visits needed per patient. However, the longer term effect (over two year period) was a four-fold increase of therapy referrals due to physician/patient satisfaction with treatment effectiveness. In addition to increased referrals, the agency no longer had the significant level of Medicare denials for physical therapy and the retroactive impact on budgeting. In describing the situation in which the study took place, most of the factors to consider when assessing philosophies will be discussed.

# TWO PHILOSOPHIES

Two basic philosophies underlying patient care were observed in the agency. One was the direct service or technical philosophy and the other, the educational philosophy. Within both philosophies the needed services are provided and positive treatment results are demonstrated, but the basic pattern of interaction between therapist and patient is quite different.

Within the direct service philosophy, the required services are simply rendered. In this framework, the goal is to improve the patient's technical performance of the therapeutic program, which in turn will ultimately achieve improved function. The patient's "home program" is designed to supplement the therapist's direct intervention. Within this philosophical framework, the patient is expected to perform the required activities as requested and to do so in a technically correct manner. However, the primary responsibility for the patient's therapy lies with the therapist. The patient in this framework relies on the consistent treatment, feedback, and monitoring from the therapist in order to maintain proper performance and to realize therapeutic gain.

The educational philosophy also provides the required services, as well as the necessary monitoring and feedback. Additionally, the therapist seeks to teach the patient and those involved in his care about his disability, the treatment rationale, and the therapy program. The goal is to instill a conceptual understanding of how the treatment relates to the patient's functional abilities and goals. Conceptual learning occurs when the patient can verbalize the principles of his treatment program, can apply them in novel ways, and can generalize his learning by demonstrating new skills not directly taught. In this philosophical framework the patients are given as much information as possible by the therapist and are expected to be increasingly responsible for their own rehabilitation. Within the educational philosophy, written home programs are a resource and a tool for conceptual learning rather than a supplement. The therapist's role changes from provider and monitor of treatment to consultant; the patient and/or his care-givers gradually become the "therapist."

## The Setting

Various factors must be considered in identifying the framework of the educational philosophy. The most important factor is the patient setting. Hospitalized patients are considerably displaced. When one enters a hospital, one is expected to assume the sick role and relinquish all control and responsibility. To expect this patient to participate in a conceptual learning experience would be confusing and unfair. Hospitalized patients expect to be acted upon; to provide direct services to these patients is not wrong. On the other hand, to expect every therapist to be able to maximally function in this setting is unrealistic.

The patient traveling to an outpatient facility has somewhat more control. This patient has been motivated in some way to leave the safe home environment and travel to the facility where direct service will be given. While the patient is making a conscious decision to travel to a foreign turf, direct service will be given and hence the patient has relinquished some situational control.

The home setting, on the other hand, allows the patient to retain as much control as desired. The therapist takes on the role of a consultant and the patient determines the extent of active participation. Of course, patients can, and often do, receive direct service in the home setting, also. This researcher believes that since the setting is patient controlled, so should be the treatment. Approximately 80% of all patients the researcher has seen in the home are open and anxious to engage in the educational approach. The others have been referred to a therapist interested in providing direct service. Confusion and inconsistency may arise when there is a mixture of various settings and/or mixture of therapists operating out of different philosophies. Some of this confusion can be eliminated when philosophies and roles are better understood, appreciated and respected among therapists.

Theoretically, both approaches are possible in any setting. An inhibiting factor is not only the setting, but also the therapist's background and need for control. A therapist who has never been exposed to the educational approach will find it difficult to adapt. Providing a patient with a sheet of instructions is simply not education. Furthermore, because the settings vary so greatly the sheet of instructions often becomes meaningless, lost or forgotten when the settings change.

The issue of control is significant for all health professionals. Physicians have received the most criticism for perpetuating the medical mystique, but all members of the health team have participated, including therapists, nurses and pharmacists. To withhold knowledge, concepts or ideas is a tremendous source of control. It ensures the patient's dependency as the health professional rations bits and pieces of the treatment plan. This is unfair to the patient. Henderson, a nursing scholar, writes that "The goal of nursing is to maintain or to restore the client's independence in the satisfaction of his fundamental needs."[1] Ideally, this is the common goal of all health professionals. Health team members need to encourage and support a patient's independence. Patients will continue to need health professionals, but the goal should be to minimize the period of dependency.

## Agency Goals

The goals of an agency providing service must be clearly defined. A therapist only concerned with providing direct service will not be happy or productive in an education oriented setting. The agency needs to take a position on either fostering independence and respecting patient goals or meeting the medical model of curing, i.e., imposing a goal on a patient. The imposed goal is often unrelated to functional or psychological wellness, but the result is often a successful therapist (or agency) since the therapist sets the goals.

Some agencies might find this decision difficult considering their desire to be effective and protective in their programming efforts. Agency directors, as well as their staffs, are frequently defensive of their own methods and attitudes. Often a rigid approach fosters unrealistic assessments of the effects. An agency must be committed to allotting time for the review of methods and the evaluation of goals.

Whenever an agency decides to be the answer to a patient's problem, the risk of underutilizing community resources exists. This is true especially for those patients who do not meet the usual criteria or who do not lend themselves to the average mold. For example, if an agency has an educational philosophy, it would need to refer elsewhere any patients not interested in conceptual learning. The alternative would be to hire an agency staff with a mix of philosophies to accommodate all patients. While this may seem desirable at first, an array of individual philosophies causes difficulties in presenting and interpreting the agency's philosophy to the community. Furthermore, this could increase the potential for frustrated and ineffective therapists attempting to work within the confines of an alien philosophy.

## Cost Effectiveness

Since health care dollars are a constant source of concern, cost factors must be critically examined in the process of defining a philosophy. Health care professionals find this concept unnerving since the basis for many of their professional motives is altruism. The agency staff must be afforded the necessary time to complete thorough patient assessments and program evaluations. Sacrifices cannot be made since the goals of treatment hinge on these two activities. The agency must also accept that quite often the educational approach decreases the total number of visits needed. This could translate to a decrease in revenue—a major concern for any agency. One possible solution is to reimburse staff on a per visit basis. They may then be inclined to make more visits per day than if they were salaried. It may be argued that reimbursement carries the risk of substandard care. Certainly adequate supervision is vital, but the therapist interested in this approach usually welcomes in-dependence and functions well.

## COMPATIBLE PHILOSOPHIES OF TREATMENT

Both self-defined and agency-defined philosophies of treatment must be considered. When they are compatible, less opportunity for burn-out and more opportunity for effectiveness exist. Kramer implies this in her account of why nurses become dissatisfied with nursing and sub-sequently leave the profession.[2] A dichotomy between a philosophy proposed in nursing school and a philosophy adapted by the employing agency is disconcerting. This contradiction exists for many health pro-fessionals; the progressive agency interested in maintaining high quality care will work to eliminate as much of the dichotomy as possible.

## LEARNING

The clinical role model for physical therapy students is an authority figure therapist, a director and "doer" of the patient's program. Fre-quently, when a home program is given to the patient, it is a supple-ment to the therapist's expertise or a mere formality. If the patient is able to imitate the stick figure positions and movements as described on the hand-out, the therapist assumes that the patient has "learned" the home program. Consequently, various assumptions are made regarding comprehension, maintenance and the home program's contribution to the total programming. This type of role reiteration can be accomplished in almost any setting; this is also not a true learning experience. Unless true learning or a conceptual understanding occurs, the program is no more than a formality. The set of technical skills is disconnected from functional activities and therefore unrelated to any goals the patient may have. In this case, a technically correct follow through is still no guarantee for an improvement, much less an attainment of functional abilities.

Conversely, once a conceptual understanding of the program is actualized, the patient is able to see the relationship between a specific exercise and the related functional skill. With time, the relationship between exercise and function becomes more apparent, and at the same time, less conscious. In fact, the functional skill itself becomes a con-tinuous reinforcement of the exercise program. Occupational therapists have recognized this phenomenon. "The therapist knows that pure exercise, no matter how repetitive, often does not generalize into daily

activities, and therefore, fails to be adaptive. . . . The adaptive response . . . is usually more efficiently organized subcortically, and, in
fact, often can *only* be organized below the conscious level. . . . We tend
to rely too much on the client's cognitive processes. . . . Purposeful
behavior can elicit adaptive responses that exercise alone cannot."[3]

## THE STUDY

The following section describes one study formulated to describe a
difference in philosophies and treatment regimes. Since the study was
retrospective, the limitations are obvious. Still, the study is a beginning
attempt to clarify differences in philosophies and possible structures to
identify which treatment philosophies are best for which setting, types
of patients, etc.

   After these two philosophies of treatment were identified and
defined, the problem of finding a way to assess their relative effectiveness remained. To accomplish this, a two-part assessment procedure
was devised. The hypothesis was that patients would improve faster,
make greater gains, participate more in their home programs, and be
more satisfied with treatment when treated by therapists practicing the
educational philosophy. A second hypothesis was that the educational
philosophy would be more cost-effective than the direct service philosophy.

   One part of the assessment was a retrospective chart audit which
determined:

   • the patient's functional abilities at initiation of services and also
     after termination of therapy
   • the rate of patient improvement, and
   • whether or not the amount of therapy was sufficient.

The second part of the assessment gathered subjective information
obtained by patient interview which included the patient's feelings
regarding being terminated from services and the amount of time spent
on home programs.

## Method

A retrospective chart audit and a patient questionnaire designed for the
study were combined to generate data for two groups of patients.
During the first year of the study all patients referred for physical
therapy received the direct service approach; this was accomplished
simply by using retrospective data. In the second year, all patients

received the educational approach. This would not be a feasible design for most settings. From each group of patients a random sample was systematically selected.

Excluded from the study were patients who had received only one visit, were younger than 18 years, were known to be unavailable for a home interview, or who preferred not to participate. The patient's functional abilities at the time of admission were determined and those patients whose initial functional score was greater than 14 (out of a possible score of 17) were also excluded. The remaining samples were: 10 patients in the direct service group, and 11 patients in the educational group (Table 1)

## Materials

A functional evaluation form for use in the study was adapted from the "Index of ADL," by Katz, Downs, Cash, et al.[4] Modifications consisted of adding three categories: "Mobility," "Home Confinement," and "Communication," which established a total of nine categories. The categories were weighted according to those functional skills deemed most essential for remaining in the home, which gave a total possible score of 17 (Figure 5.1).

A survey form was developed for use in the study to evaluate the patients' subjective perceptions and feelings about their experiences in therapy (Figure 5.2).

## Procedure

A chart audit, completed by the author, determined functional abilities for each subject at the time of the initial visit based on documentation. A second score was obtained at an average of seven months after initiation of treatment. (Due to differing lengths of treatment time, the scores at termination, while available, were not statistically compared.)

The functional skills at initiation and at seven months were submitted to a linear models procedure and univariate analysis (MANOVA) to isolate the effects of length of treatment time, initial functional levels, and treatment group placement on the patient's functional outcome.

Following termination of services, trained volunteers visited each patient and administered the patient survey questionnaire. The data obtained from this questionnaire could not be statistically analyzed due to the fact that all questions were not answered by all subjects. Nevertheless, the survey yielded important information regarding the patients' experiences in therapy.

TABLE I - PATIENT INFORMATION

## DIRECT SERVICE STUDY GROUP

| PATIENT # | SEX | AGE | DIAGNOSIS |
|---|---|---|---|
| 1 | M | 84 | Arthritis |
| 2 | F | 48 | Cancer |
| 3 | F | 90 | Shingles |
| 4 | M | 74 | CVA |
| 5 | M | 86 | Chronic Brain Syndrome |
| 6 | M | 62 | CVA |
| 7 | F | 70 | Parkinsons |
| 8 | M | 88 | COPD |
| 9 | M | 74 | CVA |
| 10 | M | 80 | CVA |

## EDUCATIONAL PHILOSOPHY STUDY GROUP

| PATIENT # | SEX | AGE | DIAGNOSIS |
|---|---|---|---|
| 1 | F | 65 | Fx Femur |
| 2 | M | 55 | CVA |
| 3 | F | 45 | CVA |
| 4 | F | 80 | Shingles |
| 5 | F | 79 | Arthritis/Hip Prosthesis |
| 6 | M | 88 | Non-union FX UE |
| 7 | F | 43 | Hip Prosthesis/Dislocation |
| 8 | F | 75 | CVA/Visually Impaired |
| 9 | M | 60 | CVA |
| 10 | M | 79 | Chronic Brain Syndrome |
| 11 | F | 82 | Arthritis/Knee Prosthesis |

Name: _____  Date of Evaluation:

For each area of functioning listed below, check description that applies.  (The word "assistance" means supervision, direction, or personal assistance.)

1.  BATHING - either sponge bath, tub bath, or shower.
   [ ]     [ ]                    [ ]     [ ]          **   [ ]     [ ]
   Receives no assistance         Receives assistance in    Receives assistance
   gets in and out of tub         bathing only one part     bathing more than one
   by self (if tub is usual       of the body (such as      part of the body (or
   means of bathing).             back or leg).             is not bathed).

2.  DRESSING - gets clothes from closets and drawers - including underclothes, outer garments and using fasteners (including braces if worn).
   [ ]     [ ]                    [ ]     [ ]          **   [ ]     [ ]
   Gets clothes and gets          Gets clothes and gets     Receives assistance
   completely dressed             dressed without as-       in getting clothes or
   without assistance.            sistance except for       in getting dressed,
                                  assistance in tying       or stays partly or
                                  shoes                     completely undressed.

3.  TOILETING - going to the "toilet room" for bowel and urine elimination, cleaning self after elimination, and arranging clothes.
   [ ]     [ ]              **   [ ]     [ ]          **   [ ]     [ ]
   Goes to "toilet room",         Receives assistance in    Does not go to room
   cleans self, and ar-           going to "toilet room"    termed "toilet" for
   ranges clothes without         or in arranging clothes   the elimination
   assistance (may use            after elimination or in   process.
   object for support             use of night bedpan or
   such as cane, walker,          commode.
   w/c, and may manage
   night bedpan or commode,
   emptying same in a.m.).

4.  TRANSFER
   [ ]     [ ]              **   [ ]     [ ]          **   [ ]     [ ]
   Moves in and out of bed        Moves in and out of bed   Does not get out of
   as well as in and out of       or chair with assist.     bed.
   chair without assistance
   (may be using object for
   support such as cane or
   walker).

5.  CONTINENCE
   [ ]     [ ]                    [ ]     [ ]          **   [ ]     [ ]
   Controls urination and         Has occasional "acci-     Supervision helps keep
   bowel movement completely      dents".                   urine or bowel control;
   by self.                                                 catheter is used or is
                                                            incontinent.

**Figure 5.1:** Visiting Nurse Association functional evaluation form. **Areas classified as "dependent."

6. FEEDING
   [ ]        [ ]
   Feeds self without
   assistance.

   [ ]        [ ]
   Feeds self except for
   getting assistance in
   cutting meat or but-
   tering bread.

   **   [ ]        [ ]
   Receives assistance in
   feeding or is fed partly
   or completely by using
   tube or intravenous
   fluids.

7. MOBILITY (Ambulation)
   [ ]        [ ]
   Independent in walking
   with or without mech-
   anical aid.

   **   [ ]        [ ]
   Walks with personal
   assistance.

   **[ ]        [ ]   **[ ] [ ]
   Walks with mech-   Does not
   anical aid and     walk
   personal assist-
   ance.

8. HOUSE CONFINEMENT - number of days patient outside of residence during previous
   two weeks.
   [ ]        [ ]
   3 or more times

   [ ]        [ ]
   1 or 2 times

   **[ ]        [ ]   **[ ] [ ]
   no time            Always nee
                      personal
                      assist.

9. COMMUNICATION
   [ ]        [ ]
   Comprehends language
   and responds appropri-
   ately, making answers
   understandable (either
   verbally and/or with
   gestures, by writing,
   or use of other aid,
   independently).

   **   [ ]        [ ]
   Comprehends language
   but needs assistance
   of a person to convey
   response.

   **[ ]        [ ]   **[ ] [ ]
   Does not           No commun-
   comprehend         ication
   language res-      skills.
   ponses may or
   may not be
   appropriate.

Expanded from "index of ADL", by Katz, et al.

(**Areas classified as "dependent")

NOTE:  The 9 categories of functional abilities were weighted in terms of which were
       considered to be most basic for remaining in the home.  The results of this
       weighting were:

|               |   |            |   |                |   |
|---------------|---|------------|---|----------------|---|
| Transferring  | 3 | Dressing   | 2 | Continence     | 1 |
| Feeding       | 3 | Toileting  | 2 | Ambulation     | 1 |
| Communication | 3 | Bathing    | 1 | House confine. | 1 |

Total of all areas:  17 points

**Figure 5.1 (Cont.):** Functional evaluation form. Scores were obtained by adding
the points of independent areas.

1. Why was client referred to our agency?

2. Type of service received:  P.T.       O.T.       Speech       Nursing

3. Seriousness of client's need on first contact:

   Very Serious              Moderate              Mild
        5          4             3          2         1

4. Seriousness of need now:
        5          4             3          2         1

5. How much of this change does client attribute to therapy service?

   All                        Some                  None
        5          4             3          2         1

6. What did client like most and least about receiving therapy in the home?

   Most:


   Least:



7. Please note the quality of therapy you feel you have received at home:

   Excellent      Good      Average      Fair      Poor
        5          4           3           2         1

8. How many days per week did you spend working on exercises or activities
   suggested by the therapist outside of therapy time?

9. In your opinion, was the type, length and amount of home therapy adequate for
   your specific needs?

   _____ Yes
   _____

   _____ No - I feel I needed:
   _____

10. Who best explained to you about your disability and why you were referred
    for therapy?

**Figure 5.2:** Visiting Nurse Association therapy services program evaluation.

11. Helpfulness and courteousness of staff:

| Very | | Moderate | | Not at all |
|------|--|----------|--|------------|
| 5 | 4 | 3 | 2 | 1 |

12. Degree of confidence client would have in referring another person in need of therapy to this agency:

| Very | | Moderate | | Not at all |
|------|--|----------|--|------------|
| 5 | 4 | 3 | 2 | 1 |

13. How did the client feel about being terminated and/or referred elsewhere for services:

| Positive | | Acceptable | | Negative |
|----------|--|------------|--|----------|
| 5 | 4 | 3 | 2 | 1 |

14. In general, degree of client satisfaction with services received:

| Very | | Moderate | | Not at all |
|------|--|----------|--|------------|
| 5 | 4 | 3 | 2 | 1 |

COMMENTS:

**Figure 5.2 (Cont.):** Therapy services program evaluation.

## Results

There were no significant differences in age, sex, race, diagnosis, and initial level of function between patients in the direct services group and the educational group. The significant differences between the two groups were as follows:

1a. Gains in functional abilities were significantly greater for the educational group than the direct service group (p < .0001); allowances were made for any differences in initial functional level (p < .0011).
1b. The educational group improved at a faster rate than the direct service group (p < .0046). That is to say, the treatment group assignment (direct service versus educational) determined the rate and degree of improvement (p < .0013) (Figure 5.3).
2. Multiple analysis of variance, mathematically combining the dependent variables of functional status at an average of seven months and the amount of treatment time between initiation and termination of service, revealed that treatment time increased, the rate of improvement decreased (Wilks-Lambda, p < .0024). Thus, the direct service patients, who were seen longer than patients in the educational group, had less gain to show despite the increased professional time.
3. The average number of visits per patient in the direct service group was 50.8, costing an average of $2032 per patient. For the educational group, the average number of visits was 12.0, at an average of $480 per patient. (Dollar amounts are based on the 1980 maximum allowable cost per visit according to the agency's Medicare intermediary.)
4. The patient questionnaire revealed that although members of the two groups were comparable in perceiving a high need for therapy at initiation of services, the educational group consistently scored higher than the direct service group throughout the remainder of the survey. Patients in the educational group reported spending nearly twice as much time in independent work on home programs (Figure 5.4).

## Discussion

The emphasis of the educational philosophy is to instill in patients a conceptual understanding of their therapy. The study results show that the patients in the educational group improved more in functional abilities, and at a faster rate than the patients treated by direct service. This could be explained by reasoning that conceptual learning is taking place. The emphasis of the educational philosophy is to instill in patients

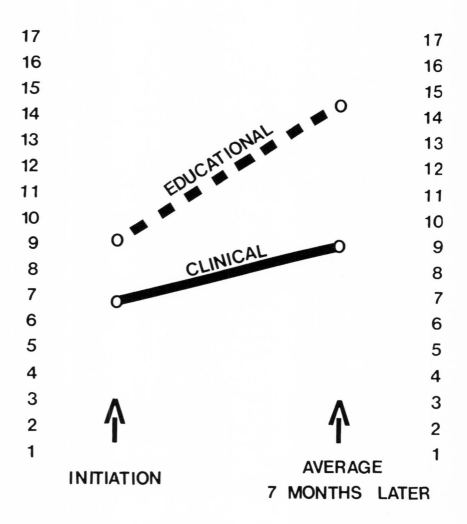

**Figure 5.3:** Average functional level scores.

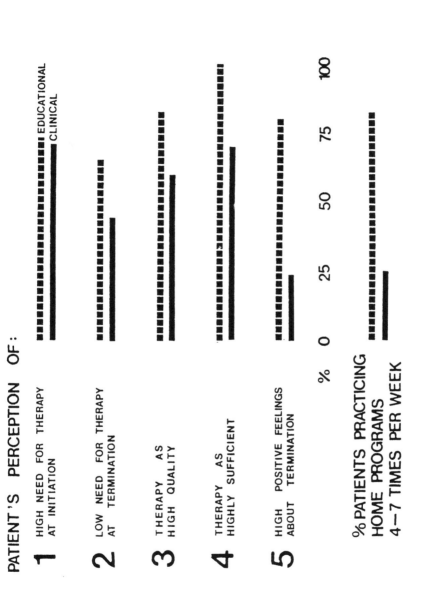

**Figure 5.4:** Patient questionnaire.

a conceptual understanding of their therapy. Educators believe that when one acquires a concept, one is able to generalize what he has learned in one context into new situations. In contrast, if one learns by imitation and rote, one is often limited to using his knowledge only within the context in which it is acquired. Observation of the patients in the educational group confirmed that they acquired a conceptual understanding of the principles underlying their treatment. They were able to verbalize their learnings, apply them in novel ways, and demonstrate new skills not directly taught.

Statistical treatment of the data revealed an inverse relationship between the length of treatment time and the rate of improvement: i.e., as time in therapy is increased, the rate of improvement decreased. If therapists know that treatment gains will decrease over time, it should assist them in deciding when the period of maximum gain has been attained. In the educational group, therapists could manage a greater caseload due to the shorter total treatment time, which capitalized on the period of greatest change for the patient. Shortened treatment time also helped prevent creating or maintaining dependency on professional intervention. The expectation was there from the beginning that patients in the educational group would become responsible for their own programs. The researcher believes that favorable results experienced early in any treatment program encourage the patient to continue and in fact to try harder for more improvement. The element of responsibility and sense of participation in the therapy plan and program seemed to directly affect the motivational level of patients in the educational group. The physical therapist was gradually able to act as a consultant rather than maintain direct professional intervention, which enabled the agency (and patient) to reduce costs. Cost-effectiveness combined with greater flexibility regarding time and visiting schedules favor the educational philosophy over the direct service philosophy for in-home treatment.

The results of the patient questionnaire also supported the original hypothesis. Patients in the educational group were much more satisfied with their therapy and felt more prepared for termination than patients receiving direct services. This points out the primary problem with the direct service philosophy, which is to convey the expectation, shared by both patient and professional, that the professional is present to do something to the patient in order to bring about rehabilitation. Conversely, the educational approach allows the patient to regain his sense of responsibility, thereby increasing his self-esteem and autonomy. When the treatment philosophy includes conveying professional knowledge to the patient in a way which encourages an internalization and a generalization of what is taught, a better chance for successful rehabilitation results.

## Conclusions of the Study

This study demonstrated that the basic philosophy of treatment does affect the outcome of treatment. When treated by therapists espousing the educational philosophy, patients improved at a faster rate and made greater gains than patients treated by therapists practicing the direct service philosophy. Patients in the educational group reported more time spent participating in home programs, and were more satisfied with the therapy they had received. The study also showed that involving the patient in his own treatment program, and teaching the family to help, reduced cost and professional time per patient, thereby allowing one therapist to manage a greater caseload.

## Replicating the Study

Further investigation into the application and implications of educational philosophy is needed. Experience with the study suggests a need for an experimental investigation with a larger sample and a treatment assessment of functional skills using a pre- and post-test design.

Since, to date, it has been virtually impossible to measure quality of care with any validity, more appropriate concepts should be examined. One example would be patient reported satisfaction with progress made at the end of the service. Another example would be therapist reported satisfaction with treatment regimes and approaches.

The study described would be difficult to replicate for a few reasons. Some of these reasons also show the limitations of the study. First is the human subjects issue. To withhold a treatment believed to be the best or to have the greatest therapeutic effect is unethical. Philosophically, the researcher would not be able to establish a group of direct service patients for the purpose of a research study. For this reason, the retrospective aspect of the described study was desirable.

Secondly, the most accurate data would come from a study using only home care patients. The turf considerations discussed earlier would definitely skew results if different home care agencies with two different philosophies (e.g., educational and direct service) would be used. Considering the competition among home care agencies, this type of co-operative scholarly effort may be impossible.

Despite the constraints, a study similar to the one mentioned could be completed. On the other hand, the crux of the problem still seems to be the inability to either define or accept a basic individual philosophy of treatment. Perhaps a more relevant approach may be to concentrate on identifying the therapist's individual philosophies while yet in training and then try to gain a deeper understanding of how best to match one's individual philosophy to a treatment setting and to patient-identified goals.

## SUMMARY

Assessing philosophies of treatment is a vital step in the "coming of age" of helping professions. The process is most notably modeled in the field of psychology, education, and nursing. The self-awareness which comes through a realization of one's philosophy, enables a therapist to manipulate the treatment of a patient to a more favorable outcome. The philosophical approach itself, as demonstrated in the study mentioned, affects the patient's attitude which in turn influences the outcome of treatment. In addition, the assessment of treatment philosophies helps to refine services by pointing out those areas in which documented knowledge has been disregarded. The questions that are evoked in the process stimulate further refinement. Understanding the relationships that exist between treatment philosophies, treatment settings and treatment outcomes is crucial as therapists enter new areas of professional involvement and consider specialty areas.

The importance of identifying, defining, and assessing philosophies of treatment cannot be overlooked except at the risk of jeopardizing professional growth. The profession's growth can only proceed as a result of the individual practitioner's growth.

## NOTES

1. Virginia Henderson, *The Nature of Nursing* (New York: Macmillan, 1966), 15, 26.

2. Marlene Kramer, *Reality Shock: Why Nurses Leave Nursing* (St. Louis: C.V. Mosby Co., 1974).

3. Lorna Jean King, "Toward a Science of Adaptive Responses," *American Journal of Occupational Therapy*, 1978, 32:432, 433.

4. S. Katz, T. Downs, H. Cash, et al. "Progress in Development of the Index of ADL," *The Gerontologist*, 1970, 1:21–30.

*Michael P. Weber,* MBA, OTR

# 6 Microcomputer Use in Program Evaluation of Therapy Services

## INTRODUCTION

The purpose of this article is to suggest ways microcomputers could be used in therapy services program evaluation. A microcomputer is a small, general-purpose computer which can sit on top of a desk. It is relatively inexpensive largely due to the development and mass production of the "micro-processor," a microcomputer's central component. "Program evaluation" is an assessment of a coherent set of goal-directed activities to determine whether previously established objectives have been met.

The uses of microcomputers in therapy service program evaluation are presented within the context of the general cyclical, goal-oriented model of organizational behavior framework. This framework has four stages:

1. *Planning* is the performance of the following activities:
   a. Development of broad goals and narrow objectives
   b. Selection of a measure of performance for each objective
   c. Establishment of levels for each measure of performance to be used as a standard for determining whether or not each objective has actually been attained
   d. Specification of activities to be performed to accomplish each objective
   e. Assignment of responsibility to a specific person or group for the completion of each activity.
2. *Implementation* is the carrying out of planned activities, including any necessary monitoring.
3. *Evaluation* is the collection, organization, and analysis of data in order to compare the actual performance of a program with the standards established in the planning stage.
4. *Correction* is the determination and carrying out of appropriate action, based on evaluation results, to bring actual performance into conformity with planned performance. This is accomplished

through modification of the planning, implementation, evaluation, and/or correction stages either immediately or during the next cycle.

Since effective program evaluation is dependent upon precisely-stated objectives with well-defined standards resulting from the planning stage, and upon appropriate corrective action resulting from the correction stage, the discussion, while focussing on the evaluation stage, will touch upon the planning and correction stages.

## ADVANTAGES OF MICROCOMPUTERS FOR THERAPY PROGRAM EVALUATION

Several advantages of using microcomputers for therapy program evaluation are: (1) they are relatively inexpensive; (2) the therapy department or a specific therapist can control microcomputer use and data files rather than central "data processing"; (3) they are portable; (4) the same microcomputer can be used for both administrative and clinical purposes; (5) they are moderately easy to operate; and (6) the therapy department or therapist can select appropriate computer programs from the great variety that is available.

## TYPES OF MICROCOMPUTER APPLICATION PROGRAMS USEFUL IN THERAPY PROGRAM EVALUATION

Categories of application programs that might be useful in therapy program evaluation include the following:

1. Spreadsheets
2. Program generators
3. Data base management systems
4. Statistics
5. Word processing
6. Graphics
7. Communications
8. Operation research

These categories are not entirely mutually exclusive. Application programs, even in the same category, differ widely in their features and capabilities. (See Appendix A for the names of several programs in each area.)

Spreadsheet programs allow one to set up a large matrix in which the individual boxes may be related to each other by a system of formulas. Changing the contents of one box can, if desired, result in the immediate change and up-dated display of each of the boxes related to that box by formula. A spreadsheet can be used to project therapy program referrals for each of the next five years under each of several assumptions for the period. Examples of such assumptions are:

- area population growth will be one percent
- area population growth will be two percent
- therapy referrals will remain at ten percent of hospital admissions
- therapy referrals will rise to fifteen percent of hospital admissions, and
- the new hospital scheduled to be completed next year across town will decrease overall hospital admissions by forty percent during the last four years of the period.

Such use of spreadsheet programs is sometimes referred to as "playing 'What if . . . .'"

Program generators are available which ask the user certain questions about the program the user wishes to develop. The program generator then writes a Beginner's All-purpose Symbolic Instruction Code (BASIC) program to accomplish the desired task. Of course, one can also write his own simple program if he knows BASIC, the universal language with many dialects for microcomputers.

A data base management system (DBMS) generally allows the development of a "data base" consisting of one or more "files." Each file consists of a number of "records," and each record contains a number of "fields." Information can be placed in the data base and then later extracted in many different combinations to meet diverse needs. For example, assume a record made up of the following five fields: (1) last name; (2) first name; (3) date of referral to therapy; (4) staff member providing treatment; and (5) date of discontinuation from therapy. Also assume that there is one record for each referred patient and that the data base is up-dated daily. A full-featured DBMS would permit one to extract, for example, a listing of any of the following:

- patients referred to therapy during any period
- patients treated by any particular therapist during any period
- patients discontinued from therapy during any period, and
- dates on which five or more therapy referrals were received.

Statistics programs for microcomputers provide an impressive array of descriptive and inferential statistical procedure, both parametric and non-parametric. Statistics packages usually contain a minimal DBMS allowing several statistical procedures to operate upon a data file that is entered only once. Due to the varying quality of microcomputer software, the user should test each statistics program for accuracy on textbook or other statistics problems to which the answers are known. Certain multivariate analysis programs such as multivariate analysis of variance and Guttman scaling are difficult to locate. This may be partially due to the limited market for them.

Word processing programs allow text such as correspondence and program evaluation reports that are entered through the keyboard in rough draft form to be molded into final form through interaction between the writer and the microcomputer. They often have powerful editing features which allow the writer to see a page of text on the screen as he deletes sentences, interchanges paragraphs, corrects spelling, inserts sentences, adjusts margins, and other changes through the keyboard. When the text is in final form, the writer merely has to press a few keys in order to print the final text.

Graphics programs (especially business graphics programs) that permit the display and/or printing of quantitative data in a wide variety of colorful or subtly-shaded forms (e.g., histograms, pie charts, trend lines, scattergrams, and three-dimensional bar graphs) are becoming readily available. Several of these programs require a printer with "dot-addressable graphics" which can print a picture or graph by combining many minute dots into a particular arrangement. Others require a plotter. (In general, a plotter draws with one or more pens whereas a printer strikes or burns to make an impression.) A minimal DBMS for organizing data is frequently part of a graphics package.

A microcomputer's communication capabilities let the user transmit information to and from other computers and their users. A "modem" is usually needed to enable a computer to use the telephone. Large data bases and computer program libraries, both commercial and non-commercial, can be accessed. Commercial data bases and program libraries charge a fee for this service. Non-commercial data bases such as those held in a hospital's main computer may be available free of charge. Dozens of commercial data bases are available to microcomputer users. Program libraries allow a user to access powerful programs, including computer languages. A program can be accessed by running it on the large computer and using the microcomputer as a "dumb terminal" just to convey information to and from the larger computer. The program may also be accessed by actually "downloading" it from the other computer into the internal memory of the microcomputer for subsequent copying to external memory, such as disk, and/or immediate use as desired by the user. Copying is subject to applicable copyright laws and software licensing agreement.

Operations research brings to bear a combination of scientific method and interdisciplinary approach to problems in a variety of fields. Frequently, mathematical models are used to help describe, analyze, and solve problems. Since the beginning of operations research in the 1930s, several techniques have been developed for addressing fundamentally similar problems arising in unrelated areas (e.g., supermarket check-out lines and hospital admission patterns). In the past, operations research techniques have been used primarily in business and government because they usually necessitated access to a computer. However, the advent of microcomputers has made operations research techniques more widely accessible. It is desirable to engage a person trained in operations research techniques to guide their application.

## INTEGRATED MICROCOMPUTER APPLICATION PROGRAMS

There is a strong trend toward integrating two or more types of application programs. Integrated programs often share a common "command structure" (i.e., the letters/symbols/words the user types to tell the computer what to do). This means that the user does not have to learn three or four completely different sets of commands to operate three or four application programs, but rather just one large set of commands. In addition, integrated programs can usually share the same or each other's data files. Finally, integrated programs generally save time by not requiring the exiting from one program and the entering of another when changing applications, e.g., from word processing to data base management. A typical combination is DBMS, spreadsheet, and graphics program. Sometimes individual non-integrated application programs written by the same firm will have overlapping command structures and can share common files. Many firms write programs as "add-ons" that enhance very popular written programs written by other firms. Both of these practices increase software integration. (The names of several integrated programs can be found in Appendix A.)

The popularity of 16-bit microcomputers has probably encouraged the trend toward integrated software due to inherently superior internal memory capacity of these microcomputers. The minimum internal memory offered in a 16-bit microcomputer is usually 128K capacity. 64K is generally the maximum internal memory afforded in an 8-bit microcomputer.

## POSSIBLE USES OF MICROCOMPUTERS IN PLANNING, IMPLEMENTATION, EVALUATION, AND CORRECTION

## Planning

A microcomputer may assist in the development of broad goals and specific objectives through the use of DBMS, communications, spreadsheet, statistics, graphics, and operations research programs.

A DBMS can be used to hold data such as authors, titles, brief abstracts, and/or key words of books and articles on planning methodology, specific areas of therapy, etc. Such an information bank could allow the retrieval of all items in the data base sharing, for example, a particular keyword, author, or keyword/author combination. A DBMS could also facilitate the retrieval of stored planning data. Communications capabilities could permit access to planning data held within another computer, either intramural or extramural. Graphics and statistics programs could allow planners to become more familiar with their planning data by organizing and displaying it in more intelligible forms. Spreadsheet and statistics programs could be used to perform "market research" activities such as forecasting the demand for particular kinds of therapy services. A DBMS may be utilized to assist the treatment team in planning individual client treatment objectives. In response to client parameters provided by the team to the microcomputer, it may suggest several alternative objectives or sets of objectives (program objectives are sometimes based upon an aggregation of individual treatment objectives).

Operations research techniques such as Markov Chain Analysis, linear programming, simulation, pay-off analysis, and queuing theory, the "Delphi Method," Program Evaluation and Review Technique (PERT), and the Critical Path Method (CPM) could potentially be used for planning purposes. The "Delphi Method" might someday, after a program is written for it, be able to garner the advantages of using a "group process" to select department goals and objectives while minimizing the distortion of the rational selection process caused by individual differences in personality structure (e.g., one person may have a tendency to dominate a group discussion while another may remain silent during such a discussion). The Delphi Method provides a way for persons to discuss an agenda without meeting. Simulation could be used to model the flow of patients in and out of therapy programs during a time period. While running the model on a microcomputer, assumptions, individually and in combination, could be varied in order to better determine the resulting effects on simulated patient flow. The Critical Path Method could be used to plan a program evaluation project. A fertile ground for both further research and software development is the use of operations research methods in occupational and physical therapy.

A spreadsheet program could help in setting alternative levels of a measure of performance for use as alternative standards, each such standard linked to an alternative set of assumptions regarding external conditions (e.g., budget level and staffing allowances) affecting the program, for determining whether or not an objective was actually attained. Such alternative standards established prior to program implementation could more equitably allow for unforeseen budgetary, staffing, and other changes than could a single standard. Alternative but predetermined standards would also tend to have a positive effect on staff morale.

A word processing program could help to write and print the plan, and a graphics program could help add charts and graphs to it. In addition, a DBMS could allow the convenient retrieval of portions of the plan content (e.g., Which activities were assigned to Susie Smith, OTR? Which activities must be completed before the end of the first quarter?) in combination and formats not provided in the written plan.

## Implementation

User-written, DBMS, and operations research programs can be used during the implementation stage for monitoring. Writing progress notes is a common means of monitoring patient response to treatment and such response is often directly related to one or more program objectives. A user-written program could structure the actual writing of progress notes by engaging the therapist in an interactive dialogue which would result in more complete and precise notes. A DBMS could be used, for example, to quickly indicate all planned activities which are targeted for completion during a particular period, are assigned to a certain individual, are dependent upon a forthcoming budget for completion, or are not yet completed. Two operations research and one scientific management technique which may be useful in monitoring the implementation of planned activities are Critical Path Method (CPM), Program Evaluation and Review Technique (PERT), and Gannt charts, respectively. The many uses of microcomputers in actually carrying out therapy program activities as opposed to monitoring it, are beyond the scope of this article.

## Evaluation

A microcomputer could assist in gathering data through the use of word processing, statistics, DBMS, and other programs. Someday programs might be written to help select both appropriate evaluation designs and statistical procedures. Word processing could help to develop and print evaluation instruments, and statistics programs could help to determine the reliability and validity of these instruments. Random numbers (or, at least, pseudo-random numbers) could be generated either directly from BASIC or from a DBMS holding many entries from a table of random numbers in order to help select sample numbers. In addition, a microcomputer can also be used to gather evaluation data by directly interviewing clients.

A microcomputer could aid in organizing collected data through DBMS, graphics, and statistics programs. A DBMS could organize data (newly collected or stored during the monitoring activities of the implementation stage) so that desired portions of it can be quickly retrieved. For example, a DBMS could organize questionnaire results so that responses to specific questions by respondents with certain characteristics would be readily available. Graphics and statistics programs could allow evaluators to become more familiar with their evaluation data by permitting them to view it in new ways.

A microcomputer could assist in analyzing data through the use of spreadsheet, statistics, communications, and other programs. Spreadsheet and statistics programs may be used to refine raw data prior to statistical analysis performed for the purpose of comparing actual performance and with the standard(s) set during the planning stage. Communications programs could provide access to statistical programs from program libraries of large information utilities. The numeric data processing capabilities of a microcomputer make cost-benefit analysis for therapy departments more feasible than it has been.

Furthermore, a microcomputer might assist in writing the evaluation document through the use of word processing, graphics, and DBMS programs. A microcomputer could be used in developing and printing the document through word processing. Graphs, charts, and diagrams may be added with the assistance of a graphics program. In addition, a DBMS program facilitates the retrieval of selected portions of the evaluation document.

## Correction

DBMS and word processing programs might be useful during the correction state. A DBMS could track progress in making corrections, and a word processing program could help generate "tickler memos" as necessary, to stimulate persons assigned responsibility for taking various corrective actions.

# MICROCOMPUTER APPLICATIONS

The use of a TRS-80 Microcomputer to monitor the completion of activities assessments on residents of a state psychiatric hospital unit is described here. The program used is written in Beginner's All-purpose Symbolic Instruction Code (BASIC). Two other microcomputer applications are described very briefly.

## Activities Assessment Monitor Program

A BASIC "Occupational Therapy Activities Assessment Monitoring Program" is used to monitor the completion of activities assessments assigned for residents of a large unit of a state psychiatric hospital. An activities assessment is a primary occupational therapy contribution to the comprehensive assessment base used by the treatment team to develop the individual treatment plan. Over 400 assignments are selected from November 1980 to August 1981. These are assignments given to para-professional members of the occupational and recreation therapy departments by means of Activities Assessment Assignment Sheet forms. A copy of this form is retained by the author and the bottom half of the original is filled in and returned by the assessor on or before a specified deadline.

Periodically, for each assignment made since the last updating, 14 facts from the retained copy and returned bottom half are placed in a 72-character "record" within the program. The program is then stored on cassette tape. A record contains 14 "fields," which represent: last name; first name; case number; date of admission; current ward; deadline; assigned to; assessment on chart, completed; assessment on chart, attempted but not completed; assessment not on chart; and admission treatment plan signed and dated. A typical program line containing a record would be:

> 20001  DATA "MILLER----------*DAISY----*
> 98765*1105*AB*1121*PS*1115*0001*
> 1120*Y*N*N*Y"

The program allows viewing the record relating to any particular assignment, or records relating to a group of assignments, on the video display in an easy-to-read format. The record for any assignment may be retrieved from the data base if the user knows any one of the facts contained in that record. The program can also provide an alphabetically or numerically ordered list of any field from all records (e.g., a list of all last names). Finally, the program can print all records in computer memory in order of any one of the 14 fields (e.g., all records ordered by case number). Processing time varies with the number of records. Sorting and printing 40 records takes about five minutes.

There is a limit to the number of records which may be entered into computer memory at one time. This limit is a function of the record length (i.e., number of characters); program length; memory capacity; and at a practical level, program execution speed required by the user. In general, the shorter the record and/or program, the more memory, and/or the slower the required execution speed, the greater is the number of records which may be entered. The practical upper limit for the program and system configuration described is approximately 75 records. Actually, processing records in groups of 50 works very well. Several runs of the same program and manual patching together of printed outputs are usually necessary for processing more than about 75 records.

Use of a microcomputer had not drastically increased the proportion of activities assessments completed on a timely basis. However, it has been very useful in finding and documenting "soft spots" in staff productivity so that corrective action could be taken.

The program described is essentially an information storage and retrieval program. It could be modified to control inventory, track residents through a hospital, organize data for research, establish a funding source data base, or to perform virtually any other information storage and retrieval function useful in the therapy setting.

## List Comparer and Sorter Program

A "General Purpose List Comparer and Sorter Program" compares two lists of alphanumeric data (letters and/or numbers). It prints in alphabetic or numeric order only those items on the first list. One of its uses is a list of admission case numbers with a list of discharge case numbers. This provides a means of generating a list of case numbers of residents admitted but not discharged during a given period. Another use is to order single lists of data.

## Statistical Analysis Program

Two relatively inexpensive statistical analysis program packages, each containing approximately ten programs written for the TRS-80, have been used. For example, a one-way analysis of variance program was used to analyze the effects of occupational therapy treatment on geriatric residents over four quarters.

# PURCHASING A MICROCOMPUTER FOR THERAPY PROGRAM EVALUATION

The costs associated with using a microcomputer for therapy program evaluation include:

- initial financial expense for hardware and software
- time required to learn about microcomputers to become an informed consumer
- time needed to learn an operating system (e.g., CP/M) and perhaps a language (e.g., BASIC)
- time necessary to learn how to use various application packages, and
- time necessary for data entry and processing.

Learning-time costs must be taken into account in deciding whether to microcomputerize the program evaluation function. However, it is equally important to take into consideration other facts. Equipment and software will usually last for several years. A modicum of "computer literacy" is almost a requirement for health professionals today. Finally, the time spent learning to be an informed consumer, how the operating system works, and how to use several application programs, may be rewarded by increased effectiveness in therapy program evaluation, in other areas of program administration, research, and clinical practice.

The system configuration appropriate for therapy program evaluation depends upon such factors as:

- size of available budget for software and hardware
- possible plans to use microcomputer for both clinical and administrative tasks
- possibility that desired programs may run only on certain microcomputers
- size of anticipated data sets
- need for portability
- importance of processing speed
- need for "user-friendliness"
- preference for color vs. black and white video
- extent to which microcomputer purchase is intended to be a learning experience
- anticipated length of time before another microcomputer is purchased, and
- peripheral devices which may be added in the future.

Features of various software packages, even of the same general classification, vary widely. Several ways to learn just what features a piece of software has are to: (1) purchase the manual alone and review it prior to purchasing the program itself; (2) ask the computer store salesperson for an extended demonstration of the program; and (3) read software reviews in magazines such as Byte, Creative Computing, Interface Age, Personal Computing, InfoWorld, Cider, and 80-Micro. One should realize that a full range of software for therapy program evaluation might realistically cost between $500 and $2,000. It is not necessary to implement a full range of software applications at one time. (See Appendix A for example of available microcomputer software.)

It is recommended that the first-time microcomputer buyer purchase a microcomputer which: (1) is "well-supported" in terms of software, peripheral device, and service availability, and in terms of the dealer's willingness to help his customers through the virtually inevitable frustrations of "getting the system up and running"; and (2) has been closely compared with, at least, half-dozen competing models on the basis of factors determined to be relevant to the accomplishment of the particular tasks to be computerized (e.g., ease of use, expandability, included software, internal and external memory capacity, cost and availability of peripherals, portability, processing speed, price, software availability, and service).

## SUMMARY

This article suggested ways in which microcomputers may be used in therapy program evaluation. Program evaluation was placed within the context of a four-stage, cyclical, organizational behavior framework. The following eight types of microcomputer programs which may be helpful in therapy program evaluation were discussed: (1) spreadsheets; (2) program generators; (3) data base management system (DBMS); (4) statistics; (5) word processing; (6) graphics; (7) communications; and (8) operations research. It was noted that there was a trend toward integrating several types of programs into one package. Suggestions were made for the possible use of microcomputers during the four stages of planning, implementation, evaluation, and correction. A brief description of microcomputer applications in therapy services was also presented. Finally, factors which may bear upon the decision to purchase a microcomputer and microcomputer programs were discussed.

## GLOSSARY

*Application Program:* A program which performs a task directly useful to the user, such as statistical analysis, data base management, word processing, client billing and other tasks.

*BASIC (Beginner's All-purpose Symbolic Instruction Code):* A computer language developed in 1962 at Dartmouth University to meet a wide range of scientific, business, educational, and other needs.

*Bit:* One "on" or "off" state. A microcomputer thinks in terms of groups of on and off states, often represented by 1s and 0s. A microcomputer that can think in terms of groups of 16 bits is usually "smarter" than one which can only think in terms of groups of 8 bits in the same way that a person who can think in terms of 20-letter words can usually understand more than a person who can only think in terms of 5-letter words.

*Byte:* A group of eight bits. Various combinations of the eight bits within a byte signify various meanings to a microcomputer.

*Computer Language:* The means of communicating with a computer. Computers understand on and off states (as represented, for example, by 1s and 0s). Human beings understand English, Spanish, German, and other languages. A computer language represents a compromise which allows humans and computers to communicate with each other.

*CP/M (Control Program for Microcomputers):* An operating system which can be used on many different brands of microcomputers. It is very close to a standard operating system for 8-bit microcomputers performing business tasks.

*Data Base Management System (DBMS):* A program for conveniently storing information as it becomes available and for flexibly extracting this information as it is needed.

*Dot-Addressable Graphics:* A printing method in which the user is able to control whether or not each of a great many small dots is actually printed. This method allows the printing of detailed pictures, graphs, charts, and diagrams.

*Dumb Terminal:* Usually a keyboard and a video display (or sometimes a printer) which allows communication with a computer by means of a modem. It has little or no native "intelligence," i.e., it cannot act as a computer by itself.

*Hardware:* A computer, its peripheral devices (e.g., keyboard, disk drive, modem, video display), and their interconnections.

*Information Utility:* A large data bank from which members of the general public can obtain a wide variety of useful information through microcomputers and terminals.

*K:* 1,024 bytes of memory. A 64K microcomputer, for example, could "remember" 64 × 1,024 or 65,536 bytes of information at one time.

*Memory:* The ability of a computer to remember programs and data. The larger a computer's memory, the larger the programs it can run and/or the more data it can process at one time.

*Microcomputer:* A small, relatively inexpensive, general-purpose computer which can sit on top of a desk.

*Microcomputer Program:* A set of instructions which tell a microcomputer what to do in order to accomplish a task. The microcomputer is able to remember these instructions so that it can perform the task over and over again as desired by the user.

*Microprocessor:* A microcomputer's central component which can hold thousands of electronic elements on a thin, flat surface about one-quarter the size of a postage stamp.

*Modem:* A peripheral device which allows a computer to communicate with another computer over telephone lines.

*Operating Systems:* A program, usually unchanged as the user switches from one application program to another, which tells the microcomputer how to perform many "housekeeping" functions, such as organizing files on disk and coordinating input and output, which is necessary for running application programs.

*Peripheral Device:* Equipment attached to a computer which facilitates input and output. Examples of peripheral devices are disk drives, printers, keyboards, and video displays.

*Printer:* A peripheral device which prints on paper. A draft quality printer uses dots to make up characters; it is usually called a "dot matrix printer." A letter quality printer produces solid characters like those made by a typewriter; it is usually called a "daisy wheel printer" due to its printwheel design.

*Program Evaluation:* The assessment of a coherent set of goal directed activities to determine whether previously established objectives have been met.

*Program Generator:* A program that writes a computer program, often in BASIC, after querying the user regarding the task he wishes to accomplish.

*Software:* Programs which tell a computer what to do in language it can understand, together with user instruction for operating the programs.

*Spreadsheet Program:* A program which allows one to set up a large matrix in which individual boxes may be related to each other by a system of formulas in such a way that a change in the contents of one box will result, at the user's command, in the immediate change and up-dated display of each of the boxes related to that box by formula.

# BIBLIOGRAPHY

Ackoff, R. L. and Sasieni, M. W. *Fundamentals of Operations Research.* New York: John Wiley and Sons, 1968.

Barley, K. S. and Driscoll, J. R. "A Survey of Data Base Management Systems for Microcomputers." *Byte,* 1981, 6(11):208–234.

Baumeister, A. A., MacLean, W. E., and Deni, R. "A Statistical Package In BASIC for Small-System Applications." *Behavior Research Methods and Instrumentation,* 1979, 11(1):77–78.

Berger, M. "Scenarios for Success: The Vision of Spreadsheeting." *Personal Computing,* 1982, 6(4):58–63.

Callamaras, P. "Executive Briefing System: A Color Graphics Development System for the Apple II." *Byte,* 1982, 7(11):164–170.

Camp, J. S. "Computer Simulations and Problem-Solving in Probability." *Creative Computing,* September—October 1978, 699–72.

Campbell, D. T., Stanley, J. C. *Experimental and Quasi-Experimental Designs for Research.* Chicago: Rand McNally College Publishing Co., 1963.

Clapp, D. E. "Queue Up!" *80 Micro,* December 1982, 333–336.

Clapp, E. E. "Linear Programming." *80 Micro,* December 1982, 70–76.

Corrigan, J. G., Bonelli, P. J., and Borys, S. V. "BASIC Programs for Two-Way through Four-Way Mixed Design ANOVAs." *Behavior Research Methods and Instrumentation,* 1980, 12(5):546.

English, C. B. "Computers and Occupational Therapy." *American Journal of Occupational Therapy,* January 1975, 43–47.

Fox, T. "Personal Software's VISICALC." *Interface Age,* May 1980, 144.

Frenzel, L. "The Personal Computer: Last Chance for CAI (Computer-Assisted Instruction)?" *Byte,* July 1982, 86–96.

James, D. "Coming On-line with the World." *Personal Computing,* April 1982, 6(4):36–155.

James, D. "Data Base Fulfill Needs on Demand." *Personal Computing,* July 1982, 6(7):32–44.

Jonas, S. "Measurement and Control of the Quality of Health Care." In *Health Care Delivery in the United States,* S. Jonas et. al. New York: Springer Publishing Co., 1977, 374–409.

Keller, W. "The Data Base Explained." *80 Micro,* December 1982, 32–38.

McGarvey, R. C. "G.E.A.P. (Graphics Editor and Programmer)." *80 Micro,* October 1982, 184–189.

Meyer, E. W. "BASIC vs. Data Base." *Creative Computing,* September 1982, 8(9):102–110.

Moroney, M. J. *Facts from Figures.* Baltimore: Penguin Books, 1951.

Moursund, J. P. *Evaluation: An Introduction to Research Design.* Monterey, Calif.: Brooks/Cole Publishing Co., 1973.

Mowrer, O. H. "Basic Research Methods, Statistics, and Decision Theory." *American Journal of Occupational Therapy,* 14(4):199–205.

Mueller, R. R. "Business Planning Software." *Personal Computing,* November 1982, 115–192.

Pelczarski, M. "A Modular Data Base for the Apple." *Creative Computing,* September 1982, 8(9):146–156.

Phillips, D. S. *Basic Statistics for Health Science Students.* San Francisco: W. H. Freeman and Co., 1978.

Poole, L., ed. *Practical BASIC Programs.* Berkeley, Calif.: OSBORNE/McGraw-Hill, 1980.

Poole, L. and Borchers, M. *Some Common BASIC Programs,* 3d ed. Berkeley, Calif.: OSBORNE/McGraw-Hill, 1977.

Press, L. "In Search of a Word Processing Program." *PC Magazine,* November 1982, 1(7):208–215.

Robinson, D. "Word Processing: An In-depth Look." *80 Micro,* September 1982, 88–90.

Robinson, D. "Word Processing Guide." *80 Micro,* December 1982, 28–210.

Rossi, P. H., Freeman, H. E., and Wright, S. R. *Evaluation—A Systematic Approach.* Beverly Hills, Calif.: Sage Publications, 1979.

Schwartz, B. "Data Base Management Systems: The New Bedrock of Business." *Personal Computing,* January 1983, 7(1):148–158.

Shortell, S. M. and Richardson, W. C. *Health Program Evaluation.* St. Louis: C. V. Mosby Co., 1978.

Stoner, J. A. F. *Management.* Englewood Cliffs, N.J.: Prentice-Hall, Inc., 1978.

Suchman, E. A. "Evaluative Research." In *Principles and Practice in Public Service & Social Action Programs.* New York: Russell Sage Foundation, 1967.

Tonkin, B. "The Creator." *80 Micro,* January 1983, 74–93.

Veit, S. "Communications Network for Computers." *Popular Electronics,* October 1982, 20(10):51–61.

Warner, D. M., et al. *Decision Making and Control for Health Administration.* Ann Arbor, Mich.: Health Administration Press, 1978.

Weiss, C. H. *Evaluation Research: Methods of Assessing Program Effectiveness.* Englewood Cliffs, N.J.: Prentice-Hall, Inc., 1972.

Wiest, J. D. and Levy, F. K. *A Management Guide to PERT/CPM.* Englewood Cliffs, N.J.: Prentice-Hall, Inc., 1969.

Williams, G. "A Graphics Primer." *Byte,* November 1982, 7(11):448–470.

Williams, G. "Lotus Development Corporation's 1-2-3." *Byte,* December 1982, 7(12):182–198.

Wilson, C. J. "Simulation: Is It Right for You?" *Personal Computing,* February 1981, 73–75.

Wilson, C. J. "Should Probability Be Added to Your Simulation?" *Personal Computing,* March 1981, 91–97.

Wilson, C. J. "Simulation: How Can it Help?" *Personal Computing,* April 1981, 29–88.

Wolff, B. B. "Strategies for Successful Simulation." *Creative Computing,* August 1981, 99–107.

Zimmerman, S. "Programming PERT in BASIC." *Byte,* May 1982, 7(5):465–478.

Zimmerman, S. and Conrad, L. M. "Programming the Critical-Path Method in BASIC." *Byte,* July 1982, 7(7):378–390.

Examples of Microcomputer Software Available

| APP | CPM | IBM | TRS | COMMUNICATIONS |
|-----|-----|-----|-----|----------------|
| X | | | | ASCII Express: The Professional -- Southwestern Data, Box 582, Santee, CA, 92071 |
| | X | X | | Crosstalk -- Microstuf, Inc., 1845 The Exchange, Suite 205, Atlanta, GA 30339 |
| | | X | X | Omniterm -- Lindberg Systems, 41 Fairhill Rd., Holden, MA 01520 |
| X | | | | Transcend -- SSM Microcomputer Products, Inc., 2190 Paragon Drive, San Jose, CA 95131 |
| | | X | | Videotex -- Radio Shack |
| X | | | | VisiTerm -- VisiCorp, 2895 Zanker Rd., San Jose, CA 95134 |
| | | | | **DATA BASE MANAGEMENT SYSTEMS** |
| X | X | X | X | Base 2 -- Xper Systems, P.O. Box 22, Dresher, PA 19025 |
| | X | X | | Citation -- Eagle Enterprises, 2375 Bush St., San Francisco, CA 94115 |
| | X | X | | Condor (Series 20) -- Condor Corp., P.O. Box 8318, Ann Arbor, MI 48107 |
| X | X | X | | dBASE II -- Ashton-Tate, 9929 Jefferson Blvd., Culver City, CA 90230 |
| X | | | | DB Master -- Stoneware, Inc., 50 Belvedere St., San Rafael CA 94901 |
| | | X | | Easy Filer -- Information Unlimited Software, Inc., 2041 Marinship Way, Sausalito, CA 94965 |
| | X | X | | Friday! -- Ashton-Tate, 9929 Jefferson Blvd., Culver City, CA 90230 |
| | | X | | The Idea Processor -- IdeaWare, 225 Lafayette St., New York, NY 10012 |
| | X | X | | InfoStar -- MicroPro International, 33 San Pablo Ave., San Rafael, CA 94903 |
| X | | | | Instant Recall -- Howard Sams & Co., 4300 West 62nd St., Indianapolis, IN 46268 |

APP = Apple     CPM = CP/M     IBM = IBM     TRS = TRS-80

Appendix A (Cont.)

| APP | CPM | IBM | TRS | DATA BASE MANAGEMENT SYSTEMS (Continued |
|-----|-----|-----|-----|------|
| X | | | X | ListMaker -- Reader's Digest Service, Microcomputer Software Div., Pleasantville, NY 10570 |
| | | | X | Maxi Manager -- The Business Division, Box 3435, 722 Commerce Circle, LIP, Longwood, FL 32750 |
| | X | X | X | Perfect Filer -- Perfect Software, 1400 Shattuck Ave., Berkley, CA 94709 |
| | X | | | Personal Pearl -- Pearlsoft, P.O. Box 13850, Salem, OR 07309 |
| X | | | | PFS: File -- Software Publishing Co., 2021 Landings Drive, Mountain View, CA 94043 |
| X | | | | PFS: Report -- Software Publishing Co., 2021 Landings Drive, Mountain View, CA 94043 |
| | X | X | | Quickcode, dGRAPH, dUTIL (dBASE II add-ons) -- Fox and Geller, Box 1053, Teaneck, NJ 07666 |
| | | X | | R:Base -- Microrim, Inc., 1750 11@th, N.E., Bellevue, WA 98004 |
| | | X | | Relevation -- Cosmos, 123 Ferntree Drive West, P.O. Box AH, Morton, WA 98356 |
| | X | X | X | Super -- ISA, P.O. Box 7136, Dept. B4, Wilmington, DE 19803 |
| | X | X | | Super Data-File Manager -- Sorcim Corp., 2310 Lundy Ave., San Jose, CA 95131 |
| X | | X | | VersaForm -- Applied Software Technology, 170 KnowleS Drive, Los Gatos, CA 95030 |
| X | | | | VisiFile -- VisiCorp, 2895 Zanker Road, San Jose, CA 95134 |

GRAPHICS

| APP | CPM | IBM | TRS | |
|-----|-----|-----|-----|------|
| | | | X | AutoPlot -- Menlo Systems, 3790 El Camino Real, Suite 221 Palo Alto, CA 94306 |
| X | | | | Apple II Business Graphics -- Apple Computer, 20525 Mariani Ave., Cupertino, CA 95014 |
| | | X | | Business Graphics -- BPS, 143 Binney St., Cambridge, MA 02142 |
| | | | X | Business Graphics Analysis Pak -- Radio Shack |
| | X | | | DR Graph -- Digital Research, P.O. Box 579, Pacific Grove, CA 93950 |

APP = Apple          CPM = CP/M          IBM = IBM          TRS = TRS-80

Appendix A (Cont.)

| APP | CPM | IBM | TRS | GRAPHICS (Continued) |
|-----|-----|-----|-----|---------|

X                  Executive Briefing System -- Lotus Development Co, 55 Wheeler St., Cambridge, MA 02138

             X        Fast Graphs -- Innovative Software, 9300 West 110th St., Suite 380, Overland Park, KS 66210

             X        Grafox -- Fox & Geller, Inc., 604 Market St., Elmwood Park, NJ 07407

       X   X        GrafTalk -- Redding Group, 609 Main St., Ridgefield, CT 06877

X          X        PFS:Graph -- Software Publishing Co., 2021 Landings Drive, Mountain View, CA 94043

       X   X        Super Chart -- Sorcim Corp., 2310 Lundy Ave., San Jose, CA 95131

             X        VCN Execuvision -- Prentice-Hall, Inc., 200 Old Tappan Rd., Old Tappan, NJ 07675

X                  VersaPlot -- Spectrasoft, 350 Lantana St., Suite 775, Camarillo, CA 93010


INTEGRATED SOFTWARE

             X        1-2-3 -- Lotus Development Co., 55 Wheeler St., Cambridge, MA 02138

             X        Context MBA -- Context Management Systems, Suite 100, 23864 Hawthorne Blvd., Torrance, CA 91604

X          X        Data Reporter -- Synergistic, 830 North Riverside Drive, Suite 201, Renton, WA 98055

             X        Final Copy -- Ticom Systems, Inc., 13470 Washington Blvd., Marina del Rey, CA 90291

X                  The Incredible Jack -- Business Solutions, Inc., 60 Main Street, Kings Park, NY 11754

             X        PeachText 5000 -- Peachtree Software, 3445 Peachtree Rd., N.I., 8th Fl., Atlanta, GA 30326

X                  The Prime Plotter -- Primesoft Corp., P.O. Box 40, Cabin John, MD 20818

X                  Statmod/Plotmod -- Blue Lakes Software, 3240 University Ave., Madison, WI 53705

X   X              T/Maker III -- T/Maker Co., 2115 Landings Drive, Mountain View, CA 94043


APP = Apple      CPM = CP/M      IBM = IBM      TRS = TRS-80

Appendix A (Cont.)

| APP | CPM | IBM | TRS | INTEGRATED SOFTWARE (Continued) |
|-----|-----|-----|-----|----------------------------------|
| X | | | | The Tool -- High Technology, 2201 Northeast 63rd St., Oklahoma City, OK 73113 |
| X | | | | UltraPlot/DIF DataGraph -- Avant-Garde Creations, Box 30160, Eugene, OR 97403 |
| X | | | | VisiTrend/VisiPlot -- VisiCorp, 2895 Zander Rd., San Jose, CA 95134 |

OPERATIONS RESEARCH

| | | IBM | | |
|-----|-----|-----|-----|----|
| | | X | | ARA Business Planner - ARA, 4040 Grandview Blvd. 71, Los Angeles, CA 90066 |
| | X | X | | Micro Gannt -- Westico, 25 Van Zant Street, Norwalk, CT 06885 |
| | X | | | Milestone -- Digital Marketing Corp., 2670 Cherry Lane Walnut Creed, CA 94596 |
| X | X | | | Optimiser -- Caxton Software Publishing Co., 10-14 Bedford St., London, WC2E 9HE, England |
| | | | X | Optimal Manager -- Optimal Manager, Stevens Electronics, 562 Nutt Road, Phoenixville, PA 19460 |
| X | | | | VisiSchedule -- VisiCorp, 2895 Zanker Rd., San Jose, CA 95134 |

PROGRAM GENERATORS

| | | IBM | | |
|-----|-----|-----|-----|----|
| | | X | | The Creator -- Software Technology for Computers, 430 A Main Street, Watertown, MA 02172 |
| | X | | X | The Last One -- Krown Computing, 1282 Conference Drive, P.O. Box 66763, Scotts Valley, CA 95066 |
| | X | | | Pearl III -- Pearlsoft, P.O. Box 13850, Salem, OR 97309 |
| | | | X | Programmer -- Advanced Operating Systems, 4300 W. 62nd St., Box 7092, Indianapolis, IN 46206 |
| X | | X | | Quick 'n' Easy -- Advanced Software, 7899 Martin Drive, Overland Park, KS 66204 |
| | | X | X | Quickpro + Plus == Futuresoft, P.O. Box 1446-D, Orange Park, FL 32073 |

APP = Apple       CPM = CP/M       IBM = IBM       TRS = TRS-80

| APP | CPM | IBM | TRS | SPEADSHEETS |
|-----|-----|-----|-----|-------------|
| | | X | | Easy Planner - Information Unlimited Software, Inc., 2401 Marinship Way, Sausalito, CA  94965 |
| | X | | | Microplan -- Chang Laboratories, 10228 North Stelling Road, Cupertino, CA 95014 |
| X | X | X | | Multiplan -- Microsoft, 400 108th Ave., Suite 200, Bellevue, WA 98004 |
| | X | X | X | Perfect Calc -- Perfect Software, 1400 Shattuck Ave., Berkeley, CA  94709 |
| | X | X | | Super Calc -- Sorcim Corp., 2310 Lundy Ave., San Jose, CA 95131 |
| X | | X | X | VisiCalc -- Visicorp, 2895 Zanker Rd., San Jose, CA 95134 |

|   |   |   |   | STATISTICS |
|-----|-----|-----|-----|-------------|
| | X | | | ABSTAT -- Anderson Bell, 5336 South Crocker St., Littleton CO 80120 |
| | | | X | Advanced Statistical Analysis -- Radio Shack |
| | | | X | Advanced Statistics -- Creative Computing, Box 789-M, Morristown, NJ 07960 |
| X | X | | X | Analysis of Variance -- Dynacomp, Inc., 1427 Monroe Ave., Rochester, NY 14618 |
| X | | X | | Applied Statistics for Micros -- Kern Publications, P.O. Box 1029B, Duxbury, MA 02332 |
| X | | | | Basic Statistical Subroutines (I) -- Dynacomp, Inc., 1427 Monroe Ave., Rochester, NY 14618 |
| X | | X | X | Maxi Stat -- The Business Division, Box 3435, 722 Commerce Circle, LIP, Longwood, FL 32750 |
| | X | X | | Microstat -- Ecosoft, Inc., P.O. Box 68602, Indianapolis, In 46268-0602 |
| | | | X | Numberkruncher I, II -- Dynacomp, Inc., 1427 Monroe Ave., Rochester, NY 14618 |
| | X | | | PAIRSTAT -- Davell Custom Software, P.O. Box 4162, Cleveland, TN 37311 |
| X | | | | Scientist - Monument Computer Service, Village Data Center, Box 603, Joshua Tree, CA 92252 |

APP = Apple      CPM = CP/M      IBM = IBM      TRS = TRS-80

Appendix A (Cont.)

| APP | CPM | IBM | TRS | STATISTICS (Continued) |
|-----|-----|-----|-----|------------------------|
| X | | X | | Statistical Analysis I -- Spectrum Software, 690 West Fremont Ave., Sunnyvale, CA 94087 |
| | | | X | Statistical Package -- A-Priori Software, 1005 West Main St., Vermillion, SD 57069 |
| | | | X | The Statistician -- Quant Systems, P.O. Box 628, Charleston, SC 29402 |
| X | | | | Statistics with Daisy -- Rainbow Computing, 19517 Business Center Drive, Northridge, CA 91324 |
| X | | | | Statpak - Stoneware, Inc., 50 Belvedere St., San Rafael, CA 94901 |
| | X | X | | Statpak -- Northwest Analytical, 1532 S.W. Morrison St., P.O. Box 14430, Portland, OR 97205 |
| X | | | | Stats Plus, Anova II, HSD Regress -- HSD, 9249 Reseda Blvd., Suite 107, Northridge, CA 91324 |
| X | X | | X | Stattest -- Dynacomp, Inc., 1427 Monroe Ave., Rochester, NY 14618 |
| | | | X | XTABS -- A-Priori Software, 1005 West Main St., Vermillion, SD 57069 |

| APP | CPM | IBM | TRS | WORD PROCESSING |
|-----|-----|-----|-----|-----------------|
| | | X | | Easy Writer II -- Information Unlimited Software, Inc., 2401 Marinship Way, Sausalito, CA 94965 |
| | | | X | Electric Pencil -- IJG, 1953 West 11th St., Upland, CA 91786 |
| | | | X | NewScript -- Prosoft, Dept. C, Box 560, North Hollywood, CA 91603 |
| | X | X | X | Perfect Writer -- Perfect Software, 1400 Shattuck Ave., Berkeley, CA 94709 |
| X | | X | | PFS: Write -- Software Publishing Co., 2021 Landings Drive, Mountain View, CA 94043 |
| X | | | | PIE Writer -- Hayden, 50 Essex St., Rochelle Park, NJ 07662 |
| | X | | | Spellbinder -- Lexisoft, Inc., Box 267, Davis, CA 95616 |
| | X | X | | Super Writer -- Sorcim Corp., 2310 Lundy Ave., San Jose, Ca 95131 |

APP = Apple      CPM = CP/M      IBM = IBM      TRS = TRS-80

Appendix A (Cont.)

```
APP CPM IBM TRS     WORD PROCESSING (Continued)

          X         Super SCRIPSIT -- Radio Shack

 X    X             WordStar -- MicroPro International, 33 San Pablo Ave.,
                    San Rafael, CA 94903
```

APP = Apple      CPM = CP/M      IBM = IMB      TRS = TRS-80


NOTE:  The inclusion of an item in the appendix is not meant to indicate that it is
in any way superior to any other product, but merely that the item was one of the
software products advertised while this article was being written.  Each of the
above software packages may be available for computers in addition to those
indicated for it because software developers continually attempt to adapt
their packages for additional computers.

*Michaele Tovar,* MA, OTR

# 7   Equipment Utilization Analysis

## INTRODUCTION

In order to ensure an efficiently run therapy department, equipment utilization should be explored on an annual basis. Analysis of equipment utilization and resolution of problems which are identified will improve the quality of patient care, reduce costs, and reduce the potential for injuries associated with equipment utilization. The purposes of this article are to:

- describe a method of general equipment review
- describe a method of more detailed equipment analysis, and
- apply the above methods.

Equipment utilization should initially be reviewed in only a general manner. This general review will identify pieces of equipment in which there are problems regarding utilization. Often general review of equipment usage is all that is needed. Results of the review may indicate that equipment is already being used efficiently within the department. In other cases, the nature of the problems which are revealed may suggest a means of resolution.

In many instances, however, such a review will reveal that problems exist, but not provide enough objective data to allow specific definition of problems or suggest a solution. In these cases, a more detailed equipment analysis is indicated on the particular piece of equipment in question.

A review of equipment utilization and an in depth analysis, if needed, will identify problem areas regarding equipment usage. Data collected will provide a foundation for planning corrective action.

## EQUIPMENT REVIEW PROCEDURE

Review of equipment within a therapy department may be easier if a standardized format is followed for each piece of equipment (Figure 7.1). This will facilitate data gathering and record keeping. A worksheet for reviewing equipment utilization and control is presented in Figure

Equipment name_____    Reviewer_____

_____    Date_____

1.  Major uses_____

2.  Results of test run_____

_____

3.  Indicate how utilization aids in achieving:

    A.  Improved quality of care_____

    B.  Reducing costs_____

    C.  Increasing safety_____

    D.  Saving time_____

4.  Rate control as follows:

    A.  Have all staff passed proficiency checks with this piece of

        equipment?_____

    B.  Are written procedures available describing use of this piece

        of equipment?_____

    C.  At what intervals have safety inspections been performed on

        this equipment?_____

    D.  If routine maintenance is being performed with this piece of

        equipment, does it seem to be done at appropriate intervals?

        _____

    E.  Describe reports of equipment misuse or incident reports filed

        in the past year related to this piece of equipment._____

        _____

    F.  Summarize staff and patients remarks regarding the equipment
        _____
        _____

**Figure 7.1:** Equipment review worksheet.

5. Costs

    A. Training_____

    B. Maintenance_____

    C. Repair_____

    D. Downtime_____

    E. Associated supplies_____

    F. Space_____

    G. Power_____

6. Frequency of Use

    A. Estimated for current year_____

    B. Prior year_____

    C. Projected for current year (if applicable)_____

7. Would increased utilization, improved control or further training yield

    A. Improved quality of services?_____

    B. Reduced costs?_____

    C. Improved safety?_____

    D. Improved use of time?_____

Summary of Problems
_____
_____
_____

Identify Objectives
_____
_____
_____

Identify Plans
_____
_____
_____

Projected date of Follow-up:_____

**Figure 7.1 (Cont.):** Equipment review worksheet.

7.1. The worksheet may be completed in less than thirty minutes. It may be used to identify what equipment is being used efficiently and appropriately within the department. More importantly, it can help identify where problems regarding equipment utilization are occurring, and what pieces of equipment are not being utilized effectively. After pinpointing where problems exist, management can then direct effort in these areas.

On the worksheet, the name of the equipment is recorded. Major uses of equipment are defined. Sources regarding appropriate uses of equipment include the equipment manufacturers' performance standards, literature within the field, vendors, and therapists' reports.

The equipment should be tested. This will allow an objective report of the general condition of the equipment and problems which are encountered while the equipment is in operation.

In order to clarify the benefits of using the piece of equipment, the reviewer indicates how utilization of the equipment improves patient care, reduces costs, increases safety or saves time. For example, use of a paraffin bath improves the quality of a patient's care by improving joint range of motion. Other examples may include the following: (1) use of a dynamometer reduces costs by providing a rapid, gross measurement of hand strength; (2) use of a teflon heating unit to soften material for splint fabrication improves safety over the conventional method of using an electric frying pan filled with water because the danger of burns is reduced; and (3) use of a band saw for cutting material for adaptive equipment saves therapists valuable time.

The reviewer also rates how adequate control of the equipment has been over the past year. Whether or not staff has passed proficiency checks in operating the piece of equipment in question is an important consideration. Written procedures regarding utilization of the equipment should be available for staff and reviewers.

The reviewer should ascertain that safety inspections have been performed on all pieces of equipment. Usually such services are performed by the Biomedical Engineering or maintenance department within a hospital. Intervals for inspection are determined jointly by managers in these departments and the therapy department. Intervals are based upon safety codes and regulations, hospital policy, and the potential for injury if equipment would malfunction. Schedules regarding the intervals of safety checks should be available from the department performing the service. Additionally, equipment is tagged when it is checked or serviced.[1]

The appropriateness of routine maintenance programs should be assessed. If equipment is serviced under a preventive maintenance program, the manager should consider if such a program is warranted. Routine maintenance programs may not be indicated if:

- the equipment is still under warranty
- replacement of the equipment is planned within the next year
- replacement cost of the equipment is relatively low considering the cost of maintenance
- the equipment is utilized infrequently, or
- malfunction of equipment would not cause injury to staff or patients, nor adversely affect clinic operation.

Routine maintenance programs may need to be implemented, or be indicated at more frequent intervals if:

- the cost of the equipment is high
- the availability of replacement parts is limited
- the equipment is crucial to clinic operation
- malfunction of the equipment may lead to injury to staff or patients, or
- repair costs were excessive in the past year.

Routine maintenance schedules should be revised whenever equipment is repaired. The reason for this is that routine maintenance is usually performed when repair work is done.

The reviewer should next record all reports of misuse or incident reports associated with use of the equipment in the past year. Staff input regarding the use of equipment should be solicited. Remarks regarding the general condition of the equipment, its usefulness in the clinic, and problems should be summarized and recorded on the worksheet.

Costs may be rated in a general manner (for example as excessive or acceptable), or more objectively by dollar amounts, depending upon the need of the therapy department. Cost areas to be reviewed are: training, maintenance, repair, downtime, associated supplies, space, and power.[2]

Training costs include costs associated with formal instruction on equipment use as well as costs associated with one-to-one supervision in use of equipment. Staff should be reoriented on how to operate the equipment at least once a year.

Maintenance and repair costs consist of costs of staff time for routine safety check inventories, maintenance department service checks, and service costs for the equipment when it breaks down. Downtime is a consideration if equipment has been nonfunctional for any portion of the year. Downtime may be indicated by a time period or by lost revenue. If, for instance, a certain treatment program required use of a particular piece of equipment, and loss of that equipment meant that a certain number of patients could not be treated, revenue lost could be computed.

Costs of associated supplies and power usage take into account the required supplies and expended utilities to operate the equipment. Space cost may be indicated by percentage of clinic space allocated to the piece of equipment or simply by space required to house the equipment.

The reviewer should record estimated frequency of use of the equipment for whatever time period that is meaningful (frequency per day, week, month, year). This figure should be compared with frequency of use recorded for the prior year, and the projected frequency of use (if applicable).

Finally, the reviewer should consider all the information which has been recorded on the worksheet. A decision should be made whether increased utilization, improved control or further training in equipment use would improve the quality of patient care, reduce costs, improve safety or provide better utilization of time.

With all of the above information, problems may be summarized, goals identified, and a plan of corrective action outlined. Corrective action usually involves developing goals in one of the following areas: developing and implementing an adequate equipment training program for staff, ensuring that equipment is safely maintained and operated, and reducing costs associated with equipment utilization.

## MORE DETAILED EQUIPMENT ANALYSIS

In some cases, there may be a need for a more detailed analysis regarding utilization of a particular piece of equipment before developing goals and objectives. This is carried out by looking at the information included in the general equipment review in more detail.

First, identification of the appropriate usage of the equipment is made. This may be done by gathering objective information regarding what the equipment may be used for clinically, when it is indicated, and when its use is contraindicated. Potential frequency of use is calculated by using these data, combined with information regarding patient population. Utilization rate may be computed by dividing actual frequency of use with potential frequency of use.* If the utilization rate is low, the reason for this is identified and the problems are scrutinized.

When equipment is underutilized, current practices are discussed in a staff meeting and problems encountered in utilizing the equipment

---

*For example, if records indicated that a Jobst pressure machine had been used 12 times in the past year for 98 patients with upper extremity edema, the utilization rate for the equipment would be 12% (12 divided by 98).

are explored. Problems which may come up include malfunctioning equipment, staff preference for hands-on techniques as opposed to using the equipment in treatment, lack of knowledge regarding equipment use, or a belief that increased time or difficulty is involved in setting up equipment for use.

Steps may be initiated to audit treatment programs where equipment is utilized to help identify problems with equipment utilization. Areas to be audited may include:

- determining if equipment utilization was actually indicated when considering treatment goals
- determining if patient instruction regarding equipment use was appropriate and adequate
- assuring that equipment was not used when contraindicated, and
- measuring the frequency of goal attainment when equipment was utilized.

Additionally, a review of safety factors concerning use of the equipment is necessary. Causes of injuries associated with equipment usage must be investigated. If there had been problems in spite of staff adherence to safety procedures when operating equipment, an attempt should be made to identify underlying problems.

Finally, costs must be explored. Are costs excessive considering the equipment utilization rate? Have repairs been required too frequently? Is space occupied by the equipment excessive when considering the utilization rate?

## APPLICATION

To illustrate the methods of equipment analysis described, two examples follow. First, the method of general equipment review is illustrated, using a band saw as the piece of equipment. Second, the more indepth analysis is illustrated using a drivers simulator as an example of equipment which could require analysis. Finally, corrective action is discussed.

### Example 1: Review of a Band Saw

In this example, the major uses of the band saw were described as:

- cutting wood for fabricating adaptive equipment and assistive devices for patients

- cutting splinting material (such as Orthoplast), and
- cutting foam for positioning devices.

The results of a test-run were recorded on the worksheet. Results indicated that the band saw blade was dull and that the equipment was difficult to use due to inadequate space.

The reviewer indicated that use of the band saw improves quality of patient care because it permits fabrication of custom made adaptive and assistive devices, which are more easily used by patients than pre-fabricated devices. Use of the equipment also was beneficial as it saved time for both the therapist and the patient. The therapist could cut materials much faster using the band saw than hand equipment. The patient could be fitted with custom made positioning and assistive devices in fewer days if the therapist fabricated them rather than ordering them from vendors.

Deficits in control of the band saw were noted. First, no staff had been formally instructed in operating the equipment. No staff had passed proficiency checks. No written procedures were available describing the use of the equipment, safety instructions, or regulations regarding patient use.

The equipment had been inspected twice the prior year by the hospital maintenance department. This would have been determined by the reviewer as adequate if two conditions had been met. First, that the equipment had not been used by patients. Second, that internal checks had been made monthly by a therapy department employee. Neither of these conditions were met.

The machine was not on a preventive maintenance program. The reviewer decided to consult with the maintenance department in determining if a preventive maintenance program was indicated and establishing appropriate inspection schedules.

There were no reports of equipment misuse in the department in the prior year. Staff remarks indicated that most employees avoided using the equipment because they did not feel competent in using woodshop equipment in general. Staff complained that the woodshop was dangerous because it was too small and equipment was inappropriately positioned. Several staff indicated that they would like to use the band saw with patients as a treatment modality, but avoided doing so because of the above problems.

Costs were all rated as absent or minimal, with the exception of space. Space costs were excessive considering the infrequency of equipment use. The frequency of use of the band saw had decreased progressively during the past several years.

The review noted that improved quality of service could be achieved in two ways: First, the band saw could be used with patients in therapy sessions. It was reasoned that woodshop projects were appropriate and indicated for patient use in many cases. For instance, woodshop projects could be used to develop cognitive skills (such as sequencing, problem solving, and measuring concepts) to develop upper extremity function, and to improve standing tolerance.

Second, quality of services would be improved if all staff could competently use the band saw in fabrication of adaptive equipment and assistive devices. Increased efficiency would be achieved because staff would not avoid using the equipment when indicated. Improved safety could be achieved by better training, improved maintenance, and closer supervision of equipment use.

Problems were summarized as:

- band saw blade dull
- woodshop poorly organized
- safety of using the band saw to cut materials other than wood had never been investigated
- inadequate staff training
- lack of written procedures, safety regulations, and regulations regarding patient use of equipment
- inadequate internal safety checks
- excessive use of space considering utilization, and
- low utilization rate.

Resolution of the above problems was handled by establishing specific activities in the form of objectives. These were identified as follows:

1. Order and install band saw blade within two weeks.
2. Organize woodshop to allow greater ease of function and permit patient access within one month.
3. Consult with maintenance to determine the advisability of using the band saw to cut materials other than wood.
4. Within three months, develop and write procedures for: band saw operation in general, use of the band saw with patients, internal safety checks.
5. Within six months all staff will have passed proficiency checks with the band saw.

The plan to achieve the objectives is beyond the scope of this chapter; thus, it will not be discussed in detail. Since the equipment was targeted for corrective action, a date would be set for another review before one year had elapsed.

# Example 2: Analysis of a Drivers Simulator

An example of more indepth equipment analysis follows. The equipment to be analyzed is a drivers simulator. This equipment consists of a unit designed similar to the driver's portion of a car. The patient using the simulator operates it as he would a car while viewing a film-strip designed to simulate actual on-the-road conditions. Responses (such as braking time, steering wheel action, etc.), are recorded on a print-out and scored by the tester.

The drivers simulator is used clinically to assess the patients capacity for safe on-the-road testing or training. Areas tested include: reaction time, comprehension, judgement, and management of driving equipment (i.e., brakes, and steering).

Use of the simulator is indicated in all patients with brain damage who desire to resume driving and may have potential capacity to drive again. Additionally, use of the drivers simulator is indicated in instances when motor control is diminished or orthopedic limitations are present. Contraindications for use would include patients with perceptual, cognitive, visual, or physical deficits which could prevent them from driving. This is too broad a list of contraindications, but more specific guidelines were not available.

The major problem revealed by general equipment review procedures was that the drivers simulator was used only two times in a one year period. This was considered a serious problem due to the cost of the equipment and the large amount of space it occupied. More importantly, it was felt that considerable revenue could have been generated had the equipment been used.

In order to verify that potential revenue had been lost, and to determine if effort should be expended in increasing utilization, the potential frequency of use was calculated.

Medical records supplied the names of all patients discharged to home in the past year from the inpatient rehabilitation service. Therapy department records were screened, and names were deleted from the list if any of the following criteria were found:

- moderate to severe visual perceptual deficits
- moderate to severe deficits in cognitive status
- the patient required assistance with basic self care tasks or transfers, and
- the patient did not drive prior to admission.

The sixty patients remaining on the list were considered potential candidates for drivers simulator testing. The utilization rate was calculated by dividing the actual frequency of use (2) by the potential frequency of use (60). The utilization rate was 3%.

At a staff meeting, current practices regarding use of the drivers simulator were discussed. Only one staff member had used the drivers simulator for her patient. She indicated that she had not used it more frequently due to the set up time (two hours) and the lack of a specific objective testing format. Other staff stated that they did not use the equipment because drivers evaluations required expertise in that area. Thus, they did not feel adequately trained. It was also expressed that day-to-day responsibilities consumed all of the staff time. They did not have adequate time to develop knowledge in this area.

Armed with this information, and considering the potential revenue lost by not using the equipment, the administrator outlined several objectives. Many were related to the general development of a drivers evaluation program. Those specifically pertaining to the drivers simulator are listed below:

1. Within six months develop a protocol for the drivers evaluation program.
2. Within six months two staff members and the program supervisor will be proficient in using the drivers simulator.
3. Within six months physicians in the rehabilitation program will be given an inservice on the drivers evaluation program to ensure appropriate referrals.

Since the equipment had been targeted for corrective action, progress towards achieving the objectives would be monitored monthly. Once staff was trained, frequency of utilization would be monitored simply by drawing data from billing documents. Staff would be informed that the equipment was targeted. Follow-up feedback would be provided to staff during department meetings regarding decrease or increase in the utilization rate of the targeted equipment.

## CORRECTIVE ACTION

Equipment review and analysis must be followed by corrective action. Often, improving staff knowledge regarding equipment will be an objective. An equipment resource book should be compiled for the therapy department. The following information should be included for each piece of equipment: name, location, indications for use, rationale, instructions for staff, instructions for patients, contraindications, additional equipment and supplies needed, necessary documentation, and common problems or errors. Staff training should be done annually and consist of an overview of safety procedures regarding equipment, review of equipment use, and a proficiency check. The focus of such training may be on improving consistency of care.

In addition to monitoring general equipment maintenance done by departments outside of the therapy service, the therapy department should ensure that all nonfunctional pieces of equipment are immediately repaired or tagged nonfunctional.[4] Equipment inspection should be done by the therapy department at a minimum of monthly intervals.

The purchase of standardized equipment should be considered in order that costs may be reduced.[5] Repair costs will be reduced if equipment is properly selected and the staff is proficient with its use.

## SUMMARY

This article provided an overview of areas to be considered when analyzing the efficiency of equipment utilization within a therapy department. A worksheet was provided to assist in reviewing equipment utilization. Areas explored on the worksheet included: function of the equipment, control of the equipment, general cost analysis of the equipment, and utilization rate. It was proposed that all these areas be grossly explored, to identify problems with equipment utilization. Following problem identification, objectives and a plan for corrective action may be developed.

A method of more concisely defining utilization rate was also presented. This may be necessary to determine if equipment should be targeted for increased utilization, or to further explore general problems identified in the general equipment review.

## NOTES

1. S. Friedman (Director of Clinical Engineering, UCI Medical Center), personal interview, November 1982.

2. D. Simmons, *Medical and Hospital Control* (Boston: Little Brown and Company, 1972).

3. H. Berman and L. Weeks, *The Financial Management of Hospitals* (Mich.: Health Administration Press, 1979).

4. B. Parker and S. Ritterman, "An Inspection Procedure for Hospital Room Electrical Systems," *Medical Instrumentation*, 1975, 9(2):180–182.

5. J. Riordon, "Rationalization of Standards for Medical Devices," *Medical Instrumentation*, 1975, 9(3):156–159.

# BIBLIOGRAPHY

Bochmueller, D. "The Management Perspective of Medical Instrumentation." *Medical Instrumentation*, 1980, 14(4) 280.

Look, A. and Webster, G., eds. *Therapeutic Medical Devices*. N.J.: Prentice-Hall, Inc., 1982.

Shaffer, M. and Gordon, M. "Clinical Engineering Standards, Obligations and Accountability." *Medical Instrumentation*, 1979, 13(4):209.

Simmons, D. "Biomedical Instrumentation Matrix." In *Quality Control Techniques in the Medical Profession*. Philadelphia: American Society for Quality Control, Annual Technical Conference Transactions, 1968.

*Catherine Erickson Barrett, MS, OTR*

# 8 Evaluation of Clinical Education Programming and Student Performance

## INTRODUCTION

The purpose of this chapter is to present information and suggestions regarding evaluation of clinical education programming based on an integration of two methods: needs assessment and use of national professional standards. Throughout the paper principles of evaluation in general will be interspersed with particular information on a needs assessment type of evaluation, with less time given to the use of national standards.

Occupational and physical therapy students at the technical level (associate degree university students), the baccalaureate level (bachelor's degree university students), and entry-level master's programs are required to complete both academic and clinical work in order to be eligible for certification in their respective professions. Quality of student clinical experiences is a continuing concern for the sponsoring educational institutions and the clinical agencies providing the clinical training.

Academic directors of allied health programs are not only responsible for the quality of educational experiences provided to the students enrolled in their programs, but also for the competency of those awarded with a degree in their disciplines. Upon successfully completing course work and clinical affiliations or field work, an occupational therapy or physical therapy student can expect his program director to certify that he possesses entry-level competency skills and should be able to pass a certification examination and/or fulfill licensure requirements. Determination of competency level rests heavily upon the clinical education program directors, who have little or no background in the field of education.

The ethical and legal implications are many. Health consumers demand competent health professionals. Allied health students expect to have entry-level skills by graduation. Allied health professional organizations continuously work toward maintaining high standards not only to protect consumers but also to preserve the very existence of the health professionals they represent. Despite definitions of entry-level competency skills by national organizations such as the American Occupational Therapy Association and the American Physical Therapy Association, there is not always agreement in interpretation of these skills among academicians and clinicians. One area of considerable confusion and disagreement involves roles and functions of personnel with associate degrees as differentiated from those with baccalaureate degrees. Disciplines seeking state licensure are discovering the difficulty involved in agreeing upon the definition of standards of competency for each level of personnel.

Some allied health professionals have begun to study field work performance evaluation procedures in attempts to establish these as reliable means of evaluating designated competency levels. Some disciplines have never tested the validity or reliability of their field work rating forms, especially those used for associate degree level students.

The importance of these standards and the rating forms used to evaluate student compliance with them at an entry level of competence cannot be over-emphasized. They are a necessary part of training professionals in allied health. In addition to these standards, however, the writer believes that clinical education programs and the students they produce can be favorably influenced by including needs assessment evaluation as part of an overall evaluation.

## WHAT IS EVALUATION?

Evaluation as used herein refers to the total procedure by which specific information on clinical education programs (or field work experiences) can be gathered, organized, analyzed, described, and judged for effectiveness and worth in order to make decisions.

A needs assessment type of evaluation determines the "perceived needs" of the affiliating student and the clinical supervisor. These needs are identified with the "real needs" as defined by professional organizations, licensing board and health consumers. The evaluation systematically delineates problem areas resulting from lacking, but necessary, knowledge, skills, and attitudes ("need state") as well as the means of attaining fulfillment of these needs ("need object"). What the affiliating student perceives to be his most immediate learning needs may not be those most pertinent to the needs of his practice, or those perceived by his clinical supervisor. The evaluation of such need states must be precise in order to make the proper choice of clinical education content and format.[1]

Another aspect of the evaluation includes defining an affiliate student's competency in terms of his ability to perform a series of tasks correctly at the appropriate time or in the proper context. This requires careful identification of situations which dictate application of specific tasks.[2]

Effective clinical education program planning and development should include procedure for on-going evaluation. The evaluation should answer such questions as: Why? What? How? and How will you know?[3] To determine "why?" provides rationale for the selection of a particular clinical education program content and format. It involves a needs assessment justifying the existence of the program. "What?" points to the program goals related to specific needs and the objectives developed from the goals. "How?" describes the program activities (e.g., hands-on experiences, interviews, and case studies) most likely to meet the objectives and the means of implementation (demonstration, weekly assignments, and feedback sessions). "How will you know?" specifies the criteria chosen to measure fulfillment of the objectives.

The types of data furnished by evaluation include: (1) *inputs* (the setting, need standards, patient/client expectations, clinical supervisor's qualifications, affiliating student's readiness to learn, content taught, and materials used); (2) *process* (teaching techniques, timing, learning style, and interaction style); and (3) *outcomes* (factual knowledge, skills developed, attitudinal change, and need fulfillment).[4] By considering all three types of data the evaluator can determine why a particular outcome was not achieved by going back to "inputs" and "process." Perhaps an affiliating student did not learn a particular technique because he did not have the appropriate background required or the teaching technique used did not take the student's learning style into consideration. Even more difficult to determine are discrepancies in perceived needs of the student and of his supervisor. For example, many students come to their affiliation with expectations that their perceived deficiencies in performance skills and knowledge will be verified by their clinical supervisors, who in turn are expected to quickly furnish the appropriate learning experiences to rectify such deficiencies. Dissatisfaction may result on both the part of the student and of the supervisor if such expectations and perceived needs were never communicated.

## WHY EVALUATE FORMALLY?

Criteria used for judging a student's competency level must be thoroughly evaluated to meet legal and ethical obligations involved. Nationally developed student field work rating forms are not available in all allied health disciplines for various levels of students. Some students are still being judged on rating forms with untested validity and/or reliability. Efficient, valid, and reliable methods (or instruments) for documenting a student's clinical performance are essential for comparing a student's performance to professional entry-level standards. Clinical education program directors have a responsibility to develop and maintain high quality clinical education programs that reflect ever changing developments in their respective disciplines. Positive results of program evaluation provide the clinical education program directors with justification of student learning opportunities and identify areas requiring improvement. Results of such evaluation can help both clinical administrators and clinical education program directors make informed decisions about existing or proposed methods of documenting student clinical proficiency and the quality of the student clinical experiences. Such information can also be used to initiate clinical education programs in clinical agencies or to seek sponsorship from new academic programs. It may also provide data for judging whether academic course work prepares students adequately for their clinical affiliations. This information could be shared with university therapy program faculty in order that course work can be made more specific to clinic needs.

Furthermore, a formal evaluation provides benefits similar to those gained from feedback in learning situations. Carefully monitoring one's behavior and comparing status quo with the ideal goal can result in movement towards that goal. Communication of expectations and perceptions between supervisor and student is enhanced. This communication results in a decrease in tension and resistance to change. In general, communication is enhanced among all involved, including the health consumers. Participants experience a sense of satisfaction, knowing that potential problems will be identified at the earliest possible time, permitting early corrective intervention.

A related benefit of ongoing clinical education program evaluation involves ideas generated for further research. This could result in investigations involving coordinated effort of academicians and clinicians working together to add to the body of knowledge and quality of service to their disciplines. Such ideas could be elaborated and carried through by students in graduate programs. For instance, one might choose to statistically correlate academic grades with affiliation ratings and admission criteria ratings. Longitudinal studies might involve:

- correlation of academic grades, affiliation grades, and 5-year or 10-year follow-up study of professional status, including job satisfaction and self-perceived and supervisor perceived success,
- comparison of recall or use of material taught in the classroom versus the clinic; long-term benefits of various clinical education experiences, and

- relationship between type of clinical evaluation feedback received as a student and subsequent type of evaluation used as a clinician.

# FORMAL AND INFORMAL METHODS USED

Prior to data gathering, the evaluator should have an evaluation plan with precisely stated purpose and objectives. It is also necessary to choose a specific evaluation design that is compatible with the type of data being sought. This in turn will suggest the required assessment tools.

A variety of data gathering methods can be used. These include surveys, checklists, interviews, unobtrusive observations, questionnaires, and the manual gathering of documents and records. Data can be organized in graphs, charts, and descriptive narrations. Checklists, questionnaires and new instruments can be designed. Although it would be preferable to statistically validate such forms, the practicality of doing so is questionable in most clinics. Emphasis should be placed on discrepancies, their causes and ability to be rectified, rather than on purely critical analysis. Explanations can be given and questions answered to alleviate apprehension and "evaluation anxiety." Conscious attempts should be made to maintain motivation of those asked to participate in interviews and questionnaires. Careful notation of perceived problem areas should be made for further analysis. Thus, comments regarding the extra time involved for interviews, filling out of questionnaires, etc., can be considered when establishing internal credibility of findings.

Time may need to be spent clarifying exactly what each of the parties involved in the evaluation can and cannot do in an effort to alleviate unrealistic expectations. According to Karn and Gilmer[5] this clarification process includes careful consideration of the following:

"Can do factors"—The aptitude, skill, and experience of the clinical supervisor, academic supervisor, and student.

"Will do factors"—The attitudes, work habits, and emotional maturity of the student; the amenability of the student to clinical training; and his readiness to accept possible "need object."

"Unable to do factors"—The rules, regulations, policy, time factor, personalities, ethical/philosophical values; and the givens to be worked with.

In clarifying these factors, a collaborative relationship is initiated in which perceived areas of concerns and expectations are communicated openly between student and clinical supervisor. Lack of agreement and unclarified expectations are likely to affect negatively any continuation of the learning experience.

The student should have some input in the content and format of the clinical experience and evaluation. Research indicates that adult learners "are more likely to commit themselves to responsible participation if they have shared to a large extent in diagnosing their educational needs."[6] A clinical education program aimed at satisfying the deficiency needs (or unfulfilled needs) of clinical education in general may fail if the program does not take into account the self-fulfillment needs of all the individuals involved. For instance, some clinical education programming in professional leadership and assertiveness with certain student groups is unsuccessful. An individual student in such a group can be made aware that fulfillment of the profession's need for leaders does affect his own individual self-fulfillment needs. Misconceptions regarding the purpose of clinical education needs assessment may have a negative impact on the evaluation procedure. This should be clarified before commencing actual data gathering activities. If we are to accept the presence of universal "needs" which manifest themselves in hierarchical progression,[7] then it follows that we accept the concept of a continuum of readiness levels. Individuals are likely to perceive needs as previous level needs are satisfied. They are also likely to receive "need objects" that satisfy various needs only when these needs are felt and perceived. There is always the possibility that needs perceived by academician and clinical supervisor may not be on the same level as those perceived by the student. For instance, a student in his early 20's is not likely to benefit greatly from a clinical educational program in "Publishing Clinical Research" when he perceives his needs to be in the area of clinical competency and job opportunities. "What is" and "what should be" are likely to be perceived differently by individuals, depending upon past experience, age, sex, attitudes, status, education, and perceived opportunities.[8] Lack of consideration of these variations in perception and readiness levels may result in student non-compliance unless clarified early in the evaluation procedure.

Inferred need states made by the evaluator may be accepted or rejected. In determining need objectives, the evaluator should carefully poll the participants for learning method preferences, rate of learning, competency variations, audio-visuals preferred, etc. Procedure for measuring learning outcomes (including those in the affective domain) should also be determined, not only to satisfy sponsor and programmer needs, but also as a means of furnishing feedback to participants.

## BIAS AND CONSTRAINTS

Bias is always a possibility in in-house evaluations. To establish external credibility, acknowledge the possibility of bias and the validity of assumptions being made. Is there bias in favor of published national standards and so called "objective criteria"? Are assumptions being made that:

- national standards reflect current changes in professional practice
- preliminary academic course work in accordance with accreditation agencies and grade point policy does, indeed, indicate that students are adequately prepared to begin supervised field work
- affiliation ratings plus grade point average furnish sufficient data to certify entry-level skills and ability to pass certification examinations and/or fulfill licensure requirements, and
- high levels of competency are the result of quality educational opportunities, including continuing feedback of performance?

Also acknowledge such constraints as limited time and budget, and the number of individuals available and willing to participate. Note that untested checklist questionnaires and other instruments may not furnish complete or valid data.

## SECURITY

Security of evaluative data can be maintained by first obtaining permission from publishers in writing for the use of all forms and data. Anonymity of interview analysis and questionnaire results must be guaranteed. Data analysis need not involve the names of individual students, clinical supervisors, or patient/clients involved. Thus, student ratings and other data can be used anonymously for scientific analysis and interpretation.

## GETTING STARTED

Mindful of variations in need perception and need readiness levels, the evaluator should validate and prioritize general areas of concern. Careful consideration of differences in needs among individuals, groups, and total system should be considered. A careful delineation of criteria of adequacy should be made. Ideally, this is determined from a combination of relevant data gathered from the literature (general norms), professional norms, and clinical evaluator's past experience. Value systems are influenced by need levels and should be acknowledged, especially if these differ greatly among all parties involved. A discrepancy at this point may indicate another area of concern which may or may not be amenable to clinical educational remediation.

The choice of methodology and instruments will most likely influence the validity of the data gathered, the inferences made, and the consequent rejection or acceptance of the clinical education program. Consideration should be given to the availability of selected instrument to measure areas of concern against criteria of adequacy, the skill of the evaluator, the time and cost involved, the environmental and organizational givens, and the students involved. The need levels of participants, easily discernible by questionnaire (i.e., based on Maslow's hierarchy) and/or interview, are also factors to be considered. If the need for job security is high among participants, assurance of confidentiality should be given and honored. Lack of security may inhibit participants from providing all the necessary information. If the need for acceptance and belonging is high, then perhaps individuals may respond as they perceive the group norms. If the need for recognition and respect is high, then impersonal type surveys and questionnaires may yield inflated desired information, whereas unobtrusive measures might be more realistic. In any case, several feasible ways of obtaining desired data should be attempted to cross-validate data gathered.

Personal needs may affect the way questionnaires, surveys, and observations are administered and responded. For instance, evaluator may insist on using a favorite evaluation instrument although participants had expressed their disapproval. This could lead to "sabotage" and invalid responses and/or biased interpretation by the evaluator. "Hidden agendas" (unspoken priorities) among all parties involved may be present. The evaluator must seriously consider the pros and cons of his choices.

The clinical education program director or designated "evaluator" should select or design student field work rating forms and gather necessary information such as academic program competencies and clinical affiliation goals. A computer search of existing literature in one's discipline and related disciplines may be helpful. For example, in occupational therapy, the following can be analyzed and compared with forms used by the clinical center:

1. "AOTA Roles and Functions of OT Personnel"[9]
2. "Licensing and Standards of Competency in OT"[10]
3. "Eligibility for Writing Certification Examination for OTR and OTA"[11]

4. "Field Work Manual for Students, Supervisors, and Coordinators"[12]
5. "Statement on Proficiency and Equivalency Measures"[13]
6. "Essentials of an Accredited Educational Program for the OT"[14]
7. "Essentials of an Approved Educational Program for the OT Assistant"[15]

Discrepancies and agreements noted in the comparison of student evaluation documents and forms can be discussed with clinical staff and faculty of the student's school, if necessary. Affiliation performance reports and field work evaluation forms of students who completed prior affiliation can be studied and discussed in order to improve the student affiliation program.

Letters and questionnaires may be sent to other program directors requesting information and/or forms used in the evaluation of their students' clinical proficiency. Comments regarding their program directors' satisfaction with the methods they use can be solicited.

Comments made by clinical supervisors and students regarding existing student evaluation forms and newly designed forms, should be used by the clinical "evaluator" and involved staff to make final revisions of the new forms. Revision of student evaluation forms based on field testing of a random sample of clinical supervisors and students would assure valid instrumentation.[16] Appendices contain sample first draft forms to provide ideas for the development of forms meeting unique clinical needs.[17]

## Data Gathering Stage

Needs are especially influential during this stage. The way in which the various instruments are administered may, in turn, influence the way they are received or vice versa. For instance, a neophyte evaluator administering his own original evaluation instrument with a great need for recognition and acceptance may demonstrate apprehension and non-verbally appear to place more importance on the instrument than on the respondent. The respondent, who also may have a need for recognition, may rebel and falsify responses. It may be helpful to explain to the respondent exactly what the instrument is measuring and why.

The atmosphere and physical set up may also influence respondent reaction. For instance, low level needs such as lighting, comfort, temperature change, rest, freedom from physical and mental pain, food, etc., on the part of both the instrument administrator and the respondent may influence the quality and quantity of data gathered. Unconscious needs may also come into play at this point. The classification and interpretation of the data may also be influenced by the needs of the evaluator. For instance, the therapist with a great need for economic security and acceptance may consciously or unconsciously bias the data in such a way as to satisfy his perception of his supervisor's need for certain type of information. Perhaps one way of avoiding such hidden agenda type influence is to use teams of therapists from several areas.

On-site visits of clinical centers by academic faculty are sometimes made to observe firsthand the quality of therapy programs and clinical experiences provided to affiliating students. Clinical education program directors can receive valuable feedback from the visiting academicians. Both students and clinical staff can be interviewed to determine their perceptions of goals and expectations and the validity of evaluative criteria. Students ready to take the certification examination can be interviewed to obtain information regarding their impression, feelings of adequacy, and preparation for taking the examination. After the examination, they can be surveyed to determine their thoughts at that point.

Notes and findings could be organized in alphabetically arranged files (e.g., program documents, rating forms, student data, etc.). Proper storage and organization of data assure their availability for future use.

## Data Analysis

Symptoms of discrepancies between the status quo and criteria of adequacy should be pointed out via statistical analysis of collected data. Interpretation of this data could include inference of probable problems or causes. This could be done by the evaluator alone or in collaboration with academicians and volunteer students. Any data that are not validated could warrant re-testing using alternative methods if any of the parties involved are not satisfied. Differentiation among performance, educational, and organizational problems should be clarified.

## Finances

Telephone calls, paper, and postage costs involved in surveying students are usually borne by the clinic. Due to the in-house nature of such an evaluation, the secretarial and staff time and service involved could be covered by present job descriptions and not warrant additional pay. Note that such an evaluation could develop into a research study with wider ramifications, thus warranting the possibility of receiving a grant or other external funding from professional organizations.

## Reporting Results

Although the original plan for the evaluation may have included only a few individuals desiring the results, more may come to mind as the evaluation proceeds. The audience may include the agency administrator, the academic program director, nursing director, business staff development director, members of professional societies or regulatory bodies, and consumer groups.

Different audiences may be interested in different types of information. The staff development director may be interested in "process data" and types of teaching techniques which were successful. The agency administrator may be more interested in the time and cost aspects as well as such "outcome data" as benefits to patient/clients. One may choose to give a series of interim reports which will include primarily "process data." Others may choose to give a final report with emphasis on "outcome data."

## CONCLUSION

On-going evaluation should be carried out until several rotations of students have been surveyed and a final analysis can be completed. Longitudinal studies of individual students' progress can be made throughout the affiliation. Individual needs change continuously as time and environmental factors evolve. Constant re-evaluation of the effectiveness of the clinical education program and willingness to adapt to noted changes are necessary for good clinical education programming.

With appropriate evaluation forms and procedures, the difficult task of grading and rating may be seen as a more meaningful and rewarding endeavor for all concerned. The academic program director's decision will be justifiably based on concrete data; the clinical supervisor will find rating more precise and objective; the student will see the evaluation procedure more as needed feedback than punishment or reward; and coordination between clinical and academic educators will be facilitated.

## NOTES

1. L. McKenzie and J. McKinley, "Adult Education: The Diagnostic Procedure," *Viewpoints, Bulletin of the School of Education Indiana University*, September 1973, 49:5.

2. E. J. La Duca and M. Riseley, "Progress toward Development of a General Model for Competence Definition in Health Professions," *Journal of Allied Health*, 1978, 7:149–155.

3. California State Department of Education, *Program Evaluator's Guide* (Princeton, N.J.: Educational Testing Service, 1977).

4. W. L. Holzemer, "A Protocol for Program Evaluation," *Journal of Medical Education*, 1976, 52:101–108.

5. B. Gilmer, *Industrial Psychology* (New York: McGraw-Hill Book Company, 1966) 617.

6. L. McKenzie and J. McKinley, "Adult Education," 69.

7. A. Maslow, *Toward a Psychology of Being* (New York: Van Nostrand Reinhold Co., 1968) 240.

8. B. Gilmer, *Industrial Psychology*.

9. American Occupational Therapy Association, *Roles and Functions of OT Personnel* (Rockville, Md.: June 1973).

10. ———, *Licensing and Standards of Competency in OT* (Rockville, Md.: 1975).

11. ———, *Eligibility for Writing the Certification Examination for OTR and OTA* (Rockville, Md.: 1976).

12. ———, *Field Work Manual for Students, Supervisors, and Coordinators* (Rockville, Md.: 1977).

13. ———, *Statement on Proficiency and Equivalency* (Rockville, Md.: July, 1973).

14. ———, *Essentials of an Accredited Educational Program for the OT* (Rockville, Md.: 1973).

15. ———, *Essentials of an Approved Educational Program for the OT Assistant* (Rockville, Md.: 1975).

16. D. L. Stufflebeam, et al., *Educational Evaluation and Decision-Making* (Itasca, Ill.: Peacock Publishers, Inc., 1971).

17. Dartnell Corporation, *How to Develop the Company Personnel Policies Manual* (Chicago, Ill.: Dartnell Corporation, 1967).

## CLINICAL SUPERVISOR CHECKLIST FOR
## EVALUATING AFFILIATING STUDENTS

Do you have clear-cut goals and standards established?

Are these in agreement with the National and/or State organization entry level standards?

Is your student aware of these?

Does your student understand and/or agree with these?

Do the student academic program director and clinical supervisor agree about the basic responsibilities and relative priority of these?

Do all agree on specific results measuring the degree to which these responsibilities are to be fulfilled?

Do all agree upon the means used to rate responsibilities, results, goals, and competencies?

Do all agree upon means of dealing with broad discrepancies in points of view about responsibilities, measurement, goals, required performance characteristics and perceived progress performance?

In preparation for mid-term and final evaluation have you –

1. Reviewed agreed-to goals?
2. Reviewed agreed-to means of measurement and rating systems?
3. Reviewed student's agreed-to "specific results"?
4. Answered the student's questions and/or given sufficient feedback?
5. Prepared the student for the evaluation (purpose, procedure, "rules")?
6. Provided student with sufficient time to fill "Roles and Functions Evaluator" form prior to evaluation meeting? (Appendix C)
7. filled out the above form?

During the evaluation –

1. Did you emphasize the person and not the grading?
2. Did you explain the finality of the ratings without apology but emphasize your desire for mutuality of ratings?
3. Did you convey confidence in your findings?
4. Did you allow the student sufficient time to read and ask questions regarding the content of the "Roles and Functions Evaluator" form you filled out?
5. Did you carefully read the student's version?
6. Did you analyze with the student major discrepancies and disagreements?
7. Did you isolate performance discrepancies without criticizing or condemning?

8. Did you test the student's awareness of goals and standards not attained?
9. Did you test the student's perception of his performance if different from yours?
10. Did you test the impact of situational factors upon the student's performance and check out whether these are unavoidable or can be eliminated?
11. Did you test the student's abilities (knowledge, skills, traits) which may have influenced his performance and check out whether training would yield sufficient improvement?
12. Did you test the motivation of the student by asking what he gains by doing; what he loses by not doing; what he gains by not doing; and what he loses by doing?
13. Did you and the student develop a plan for action? (provision for additional guidance, training, and means for reviewing?)

Appendix B

National organization published roles and functions are usually stated in
several terms.  Individual clinical affiliation center differences are not
reflected.

The following questionnaire could be filled out by clinical supervisor, student,
and academic program director.  Results could be compared in an effort to come
to some mutual agreement regarding entry level responsibilities and performance
characteristics needed within a particluar setting and in accordance with
national (and possibly state) standards.  NOTE - They can be answered as pertaining
to entry-level staff or beginning affiliating students.

---

PERFORMANCE CHARACTERISTICS
OF ENTRY-LEVEL TECHNICAL STATE*

AFFILIATION CENTER_____ Date:_____

EVALUATOR:_____

Describe below the most important personal requirements for an entry-
level staff (or beginning affiliating student) in this setting in the
categories shown.

1.  What are the most important kinds of knowledge needed, such as
    knowledge of wheelchairs, anatomy, developmental stages, psychi-
    atric signs and symptoms?

2.  What are the most important kinds of skills to have, such as plan-
    ning skills, leadership ability, writing, problem-solving, deci-
    sion-making, verbal. etc.?

3.  What are the most important traits to have, such as self-confi-
    dence, assertiveness, empathy, patience, creativity, etc.?

---

*Adapted from Darnell Corporation "JOB EVALUATOR"

149

Appendix C

ROLES AND FUNCTIONS EVALUATOR

| Responsibilities | Measurement | Perceived Progress | Goals |
|---|---|---|---|
| List in order of importance the major responsibilities entry-level staff. (Use as few words as possible such as "interview patients", "do inventory", "lead re-motivation group", ect.) | For each responsibility shown, state the result that can be seen or measured that indicate how well the responsibility has been carried out. (Such as, "initial note", "test results", "treatment plan".) List as many results as appropriate for each responsibility. | How well is each of these results being carried out? (Give a numerical rating for each result where<br>4 = being exceeded<br>3 = being generally met<br>2 = initially (or some) met<br>1 = not met at all<br>0 = do not know | Below describe briefly any special goals or projects being worked on, over and above normal responsibilities. (Such as decorating bulletin boards, creating a new adaptive equipment, etc.) |
| 1. | | | |
| 2. | | | |
| 3. | | | |
| 4. | | | |
| 5. | | | |
| 6. | | | |
| 7. | | | |
| 8. | | | |
| 9. | | | |
| 10. | | | |
| 11. | | | |
| 12. | | | |

Adapted from Dartnell Corporation "JOB EVALUATOR"

Appendix D

---

STUDENT'S MID-TERM PLANNING
WORKSHEET

1. State below exactly what help you will require to carry out your
   plans including what this help consists of, and how you believe
   it should be provided.




2. State below the rate of progress you feel is reasonable in
   achieving part results, goals, etc.  That is, how much progress
   should have occurred by what time?




3. Indicate below your preferred times for feedback sessions for
   the duration of your affiliation.



---

The above form could be filled out by the student just prior to mid-term
evaluation.  The results shared with the clinical supervisor could be
used to correct faulty perceptions and/or expectations and to make
necessary adjustments or to validate them.